FAST FACTS FOR CURRICULUM DEVELOPMENT IN NURSING

Janice L. McCoy, PhD, RN, held early career roles as a school nurse, flight nurse, and cardiac catheterization lab nurse. For the majority of her nursing career, she held appointments at Central Wyoming College, as nursing faculty, as nursing program director, division chair, Professional/Technical Division (1990–1993) and Allied Health Division (1993–1999), and as director of Distance Education/Lifelong Learning (1999–2002).

More recently, Dr. McCoy has served as nursing faculty at Walden University; individual service coordinator, Wyoming Department of Health; independent contractor and consultant for Sylvan Learning Systems; as well as interim director of nursing programs and mentor, Western Governors University, Salt Lake City, Utah.

She holds an online instructor certificate from Walden University and was awarded a Kellogg Fellowship through the University of Portland.

Marion G. Anema, PhD, RN, most recently served as educational resources director (a joint position with Mid America Learning and Texas Education Resources) to consult and develop distance education programs with institutional partners. She was also chief academic officer at Mid America Learning managing and implementing nursing programs with institutional partners.

Dr. Anema has held administrative and faculty positions as associate director, Nursing Programs, College of Health Professions, Western Governors University; faculty chair, Walden University; dean, School of Nursing, Tennessee State University; and assistant dean, Texas Woman's University, Dallas.

She holds certificates as an online instructor in case management, online quality management, and intensive bioethics (Georgetown University). Her scholarly articles have been published in *Dimensions of Critical Care Nursing, Journal of Nursing Administration, Nursing, Journal of Nursing Education, Nurse Educator, International Nursing Review, Computers in Nursing,* and *Journal of Continuing Education in Nursing,* among others.

Dr. McCoy and Dr. Anema published *Competency-Based Nursing Education: Guide to Achieving Outstanding Learner Outcomes* in 2010 (Springer Publishing Company). They continue to provide consulting services for nursing programs involved in curriculum development/revision and/or program accreditation processes.

FAST FACTS FOR CURRICULUM DEVELOPMENT IN NURSING

How to Develop & Evaluate Educational Programs in a Nutshell

Janice L. McCoy, PhD, RN

Marion G. Anema, PhD, RN

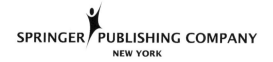

SPRINGER PUBLISHING COMPANY

NEW YORK

Springer Publishing Company, LLC
11 West 42nd Street
New York, NY 10036
www.springerpub.com

Acquisitions Editor: Margaret Zuccarini
Composition: S4Carlisle Publishing Services

ISBN: 978-0-8261-0998-9
E-book ISBN: 978-0-8261-0999-6

12 13 14/ 5 4 3 2 1

The author and the publisher of this Work have made every effort to use sources believed to be reliable to provide information that is accurate and compatible with the standards generally accepted at the time of publication. The author and publisher shall not be liable for any special, consequential, or exemplary damages resulting, in whole or in part, from the readers' use of, or reliance on, the information contained in this book. The publisher has no responsibility for the persistence or accuracy of URLs for external or third-party Internet Web sites referred to in this publication and does not guarantee that any content on such Web sites is, or will remain, accurate or appropriate.

Library of Congress Cataloging-in-Publication Data

McCoy, Janice L.
  Fast facts for curriculum development in nursing: how to develop & evaluate educational programs in a nutshell/Janice L. McCoy, Marion G. Anema.
    p. ; cm.
  Includes bibliographical references and index.
  ISBN-13: 978-0-8261-0998-9
  ISBN-10: 0-8261-0998-5
  ISBN-13: 978-0-8261-0999-6 (e-book)
  I. Anema, Marion G. II. Title.
    [DNLM: 1. Education, Nursing. 2. Curriculum. 3. Nursing Evaluation
    Research.   WY 18]
  Lc classification not assigned
  610.72—dc23
                                                                        2012006094

Printed in the United States of America by Hamilton Printing

Contents

Part III: Curriculum and Course Design

Part IV: Evaluation of Programs and Curricula

Preface

The primary purpose of this book is to guide nurse educators through the challenging process of developing and evaluating educational offerings, whether at the program level or the individual course level. It is predicted that demands on the health care system will require additional nurses at all levels of preparation. Increased demands on the health care system will also require an increase in patient education courses, with the goal of assisting consumers to become knowledgeable about maintaining their own health. The responsibilities for maintaining and improving individual health must be shared between the nurse and the consumer. Professional groups need to determine best practices and evidence, informed consumers need to know how to care for themselves, and health providers need to be prepared to provide the needed education.

Rapidly changing practice standards and advances in health care technology require informed and competent health care providers; thus, staff developers need to develop and evaluate continuing education offerings. Many nurses entering the educational environment come directly from clinical practice. While very knowledgeable about current practice standards and expectations, these new educators are unfamiliar with the program and course development requirements and educational standards. The bottom line is that all health care providers are educators and need to be aware of the accepted standards for development and evaluation of all health education offerings. While textbooks explaining the program or curricular processes abound, this book is designed as a "how-to" book to quickly guide the novice educator in the development of programs or courses that meet most approval/accrediting agency standards. The book can be used to create new programs or courses, and it can also be used to revise existing programs and courses. It does not stop with the development process but includes an evaluation process so decisions can be based on data. The book emphasizes that data collection is not sufficient if data analysis does not occur, and provides examples to assist the educator in data analysis, the transforming of data into information for decision-making. The book also includes suggestions on how to transform the curriculum, programs, and individual educational offerings into competency-based educational systems.

This book is divided into four parts. Part I consists of five chapters and follows a step-by-step process especially helpful in developing all types of nursing education programs. Part I provides a summary of nursing program approval/accreditation processes and stresses the importance of using systems thinking in program development. In addition, Part I explains how to develop the program elements required by many approval/accrediting agencies.

Chapter 1 summarizes the processes for program approval at the local and state levels. Considerations for making national accreditation decisions are incorporated. Chapter 2 reviews the basic concepts and principles of systems thinking. Program and course development can be simplified when approached through the lens of systems. Chapter 3 begins with the development of a mission statement that is congruent with the mission of the organization/parent institution. Chapter 4 moves on to the development of a program philosophy that is congruent with the philosophy of the organization/parent institution. The development of a program philosophy statement explains how the program mission is achieved. Chapter 5 discusses the development of an organizing framework. It is from the program philosophy statement and the organization/parent institution required learner attributes that the major concepts are identified and defined.

Part II consists of four chapters that build on the Part I chapters and guide the development of educational and level outcomes as well as curricular mapping processes. The importance for faculty to accept responsibility for program/curricular development is emphasized.

Chapter 6 guides the reader in the development of educational outcomes. Educational outcomes delineate what learners need to know and to be able to do at the completion of the program or educational offering. Chapter 7 takes the educational outcomes and levels them either by program level or by end-of-semester expectations or educational offering. Leveling assists educators in selecting or designing educational experiences that are at an appropriate learning level and demonstrate progression. Chapter 8 explains curriculum mapping of the concepts and subconcepts from the organizing framework to ensure all concepts are present, leveled appropriately, and progress from simpler expectations to more complex expectations. Curriculum mapping also guides educators with course development so educational experiences are at an appropriate level and demonstrate progression, reduce duplication, and minimize gaps. Chapter 9 discusses the important role that faculty play in program development or revision. Preparing faculty for new roles and the changes that are required are presented. Strategies to overcome resistance to change are also included. Successful program development or revision is dependent on willing and committed faculty. Part III consists of three chapters addressing curriculum and course design using an organizing framework.

Chapter 10 summarizes the elements of a curriculum and the importance of incorporating the program philosophy and organizing framework. Several factors that influence curriculum development are included. Chapter 11 presents a variety of curriculum design and delivery options, as well as a variety of organizing structures that support curriculum design. Chapter 12 summarizes several options for course design to meet institutional, educational, and professional requirements. Different types of teaching strategies are considered.

Part IV consists of five chapters and addresses evaluation processes. Part IV pulls everything together in the evaluation of programs and curriculum.

Chapter 13 discusses the identification of program outcomes. Where educational outcomes specify what the learner is expected to demonstrate at program completion, program outcomes identify the expectations for the program and are often reported as aggregate data.

Chapter 14 pulls all the previous elements together in a comprehensive, systematic evaluation process. The evaluation process begins when a program or course is first developed or revised. Data about the effectiveness and quality of the education offering are collected and analyzed, thus allowing for trended data over time—semester, year, or multiple years. Chapter 15 focuses on assessing program outcomes to determine if goals have been met and to support changes for individual courses and learners, relating level of achievement to program and organizational benchmarks. Chapter 16 examines the curriculum data related to individual learners and courses. The outcome is compared to the expected levels of achievement and benchmarks for the program. Chapter 17 examines the processes for using program and course outcome data to analyze and review programs. The goal is to improve programs.

Changing current educational programs and courses or developing new ones can be done using the different chapter information as needed. It is not usually necessary to change entire programs or courses. The Internet is a rich resource for similar types of information, samples of documents and reports, and examples of educational offerings based on best practices.

Janice L. McCoy
Marion G. Anema

FAST FACTS FOR CURRICULUM DEVELOPMENT IN NURSING

Nursing Program Foundations

I

Considerations When Starting or Revising Nursing Programs

INTRODUCTION

Before implementing a new nursing educational program or making major changes to an existing program, several approval requirements must be met. Every organization has an approval process for new programs or major changes in an existing program and this process will differ from one organization to another. Once a nursing program, new or revised, has organizational approval, the next step is to secure state approval. Typically, this state approval is granted through the board of nursing, but other state agencies may be involved. The next step in the process may be achieving national accreditation. Usually a new nursing program must have students enrolled before national accreditation can be initiated. Each program level (practical nursing, associate degree, baccalaureate) must meet specified program standards: organization, state board of nursing, and accrediting agency. Prior planning for new nursing program approval is essential since it can take up to one year to implement the program. Knowledge about the approval processes and specific program requirements will aid program development and implementation.

In this chapter, you will learn:

1. What to consider when seeking approval for a new nursing program or major revisions to an existing program within an organization.
2. What to consider when seeking approval for a new nursing program or major revisions to an existing program from state regulatory agencies.
3. What to consider when seeking accreditation for a new nursing program or major revisions to an existing program from a national accrediting agency.

PURPOSES FOR NURSING PROGRAM APPROVAL AND ACCREDITATION PROCESSES

The goals for new nursing programs depend on the organization or agency involved. Educational institutions use the internal approval process to determine if the new program is congruent with the instutional mission and if the program will further that mission. Educational institutions also have internal standards for program quality and proposed programs must demonstrate adherence to institutional educational standards. In addition, educational institutions must have the necessary resources available to support the new program and must evaluate what resources are required and if they are available. Extensive revisions of an existing program may require institutional approval but the process may not be as extensive as with new programs.

State boards of nursing are charged with protecting the public; one way they accomplish this charge is through the nursing program approval and continued approval processes. Most state boards of nursing establish and publish standards of nursing practice and review new and existing nursing programs for the graduates' ability to practice within standards. In addition, state boards of nursing determine program quality using established and published educational standards. The program standards are applied to requests for new programs as well as existing programs.

Like state boards of nursing, national accrediting agencies have published nursing education standards. Achieving national accreditation means the program has met or exceeded the standards for quality nursing education.

Definition of Key Terms
- **Approval** is a written consent by a regulatory body to proceed with a requested activity; an official agreement or permission, given by someone in authority based on meeting a minimum set of regulations.
- **Accreditation** means granting of approval to an institution of learning by an official review board after the school has met specific requirements. It is a process of formal recognition of a school or institution attesting to the required ability and performance in an area of education, training, or practice.
- **Educational accreditation** is a type of quality assurance process under which an external body evaluates the services and operations of educational institutions or programs, determining if applicable standards have been met.

KEY POINTS

Internal

Educational institutions usually have in place a defined process for approving new programs. This process will differ from institution to institution. Securing institutional approval is the first step in offering a new nursing program. Be prepared to allocate up to one year for the internal approval process to complete its course. Typically, proposals for new programs are formal documents, include specific and defined requirements, and must be approved by the institution administration and their governing board.

State

In addition to new nursing program approval from the appropriate state board of nursing, there may also be a state education board or commission that must approve all new programs. The education boards or commissions publish the requirements and will vary from state to state. You can find a link to your state board of nursing on the National Council of State Boards of Nursing (NCSBN, 2011) website.

State boards of nursing establish the requirements for new program approval. These requirements are typically published in their administrative rules and regulations. Individual state board of nursing program requirements can be found using the National Council of State Boards of Nursing (NCSBN, 2011) website.

Since there are multiple entry levels for nurses, programs must designate which entry level will be offered and incorporate the appropriate educational and practice standards. The following nursing organizations publish supplemental information that can assist in program development.

- National Association for Practical Nurse Education and Service (NAPNES, 2007)
- National Organization for Associate Degree Nursing (NOADN, 2006)
- American Association of Colleges of Nursing [baccalaureate and master's] (AACN, 2008)

State boards of nursing also have a defined process for continuing approval of existing nursing programs. Continuing approval processes can be found in the state boards of nursing administrative rules and regulations and typically require the submission of a self-study document, addressing the individual state board of nursing educational standards. An onsite visit is usually required, where representatives of the state board of nursing verify the self-study documentation.

≡FAST FACTS in a NUTSHELL

Program approval at the local and state levels is mandatory for all new nursing programs.

National

Many educators consider national accreditation desirable for nursing programs. The two organizations accrediting nursing programs are the National League for Nursing Accrediting Commission (NLNAC) and the Commission on Collegiate Nursing Education (CCNE). The agency chosen will sometimes depend on the type of program offered. NLNAC accredits practical nursing, associate degree, baccalaureate, and master's degree programs. CCNE accredits baccalaureate, master's, and doctorate of nursing practice degree programs. If the new program is at the baccalaureate degree or higher, either accrediting agency may be used. Both accrediting organizations publish standards that must be addressed in a formal self-study document and verified through an onsite visit.

Timing of initial accreditation has implications for students/graduates. NLNAC considers all students who graduated during accreditation cycle when the site visit was performed to be graduates of an accredited nursing program. CCNE considers only those students who graduate after accreditation has been granted to be graduates of an accredited nursing program.

≡FAST FACTS in a NUTSHELL

Accreditation is a voluntary method of quality assurance.

EXAMPLES OF NURSING PROGRAM APPROVAL PROCESSES

Internal

Typically, new nursing programs are initiated in conjunction with faculty and academic administrators. The need for the program must be established and is usually accomplished through a needs assessment. Once the need for the program has been established, a detailed proposal is written. While each institution has specific proposal requirements, the following are fairly common.

- Description of the new program
- Purpose of the new program
- Clear evidence of a need for the new program, with supporting data (needs assessment)
- Program content and quality
- Plan for periodic evaluation of program effectiveness
- Necessary resources and support for the new program
- Projected enrollment and student costs

FAST FACTS in a NUTSHELL

If possible, address the state board of nursing requirements for new program approval into the proposal submitted for internal approval. Doing so will save time.

The completed new program proposal is submitted through the established institutional approval channels. Once approved by the institution and the local governing board, the approval process moves to the state level.

State

The next step is approval from the state education board/commission or other pertinent body. The proposal developed for the institution is commonly used to acquire this level of approval but there may be additional forms to be completed. Once the state education board/commission or other pertinent body approves the program, a new program proposal is submitted to the state board of nursing. Boards of nursing publish the requirements and process for new program approval in their administrative rules and regulations.

Proposals submitted to the board of nursing may require similar information requested at the local level. The following are examples of board of nursing proposal requirements:

- Evidence of approval from the pertinent governing body, state education board, or commission
- Rationale for establishing a new nursing education program, including need for present/future entry-level nurses in the state and potential effects on other nursing programs in the state
- Relationship of the nursing education program within the institution
- Purpose, mission, and level of the proposed nursing education program
- Evidence of adequate resources for planning, implementation, and continuation of the program
- Anticipated student populations

Provisional approval from the board of nursing must be granted before students can be admitted to a new program. Once the new program is populated with students, the program must complete a self-study document and schedule an onsite visit before full approval is granted. State boards of nursing have timelines specifying when the full approval process must occur.

National

Once full approval has been granted by the state board of nursing, the decision to seek national accreditation can be made. National accreditation is accomplished through one of two accrediting agencies (NLNAC or CCNE), and the selection will depend on program type or preference. Timing of the accreditation cycle must also be considered to afford graduates the benefits of graduating from an accredited program. Both organizations have a formal application process. Similar to the internal and state approval processes, there are published standards that must be addressed. NLNAC (2008) has six standards, while CCNE (2009) has four. Although the standards are organized slightly differently, they address similar areas. The standards are used to direct the creation of the formal self-study document and prepare the program for the onsite visit. Table 1.1 lists the broad standards categories for NLNAC and CCNE.

TABLE 1.1 NLNAC and CCNE Program Standards

NLNAC Program Standards	CCNE Program Standards
Mission and administrative capacity	Program quality: mission and governance
Faculty and staff	Program quality: curriculum and teaching-learning practices
Students	Program quality: institutional commitment and resources
Curriculum	
Resources	Program effectiveness: aggregate student and faculty outcomes
Outcomes	

The decision to start a new nursing program should not be taken lightly. There are many steps in the approval and accreditation processes, and they require substantial work in order to move through the many local, state, and national layers. The following chapters should assist in the development of the necessary documents for successful program revisions or new program creation.

2

Overview of Systems Thinking

INTRODUCTION

Applying the concepts and principles of systems thinking adds to the understanding that all parts of a program are connected. One common characteristic of all systems is that knowing one part of a system enables us to know something about another part. Understanding the interactions within a curricular system is important because a change in one component of a program may induce a change in another component. Likewise, understanding interdependence within a curricular system demonstrates where a change in one component may induce a change in another component.

In this chapter, you will learn:

1. How systems thinking applies the basic concepts and principles from systems theory.
2. How systems thinking can guide nurse educators in the development of educational programs.
3. Why it is important to focus on the whole educational program instead of the individual program components.

PURPOSES OF SYSTEMS THINKING

Systems thinking is based on systems theory. The main function of systems theory is to provide a theoretical model for explaining, predicting, and controlling phenomena. Systems theory surfaced as an attempt to identify the characteristics common to all systems. Nurses are familiar with systems theory through the study of the human body.

Systems thinking is a process that applies the common characteristics identified in systems theory to the whole system (Leischow & Milstein, 2006). Systems thinking focuses on the big picture—the whole program rather than the individual elements of the program. Systems thinking helps to create solutions and avoid undue focus on effects resulting from causes that may be part of another system altogether.

Definition of Key Terms
- **Systems** are organized as wholes composed of component parts that interact in a distinct way over time.
- **General systems theory** suggests that all systems, regardless of their type or level of organization, share certain characteristics that allow them to function as systems.
- **Systems thinking** is the process of conceptualizing changes in the context of the total system.

KEY POINTS

Systems thinking has its roots in general system theory. General systems theory focuses on the system's structure and how that structure can impact a system's function. Systems theory proposes that complex systems share some basic organizing principles regardless of the purpose of the system.

FAST FACTS in a NUTSHELL

Shared Organizing Principles of Systems Theory

- Systems are subsystems of larger systems.
- Real systems are open to, and interact with, their internal and external environments.
- Emphasis is placed on the interrelatedness and mutual interdependence of all the elements of a system.
- Program elements cannot be understood in isolation but must be seen as part of a system.
- Systems adjust in order to maintain balance.

While general systems theory initially addressed biological systems, over time it has evolved to be applicable to many fields of study. Hospitals are structured using the general organizing principles from systems theory. A typical hospital structure includes many internal subsystems, such as nursing, pharmacy, dietary, outpatient services, surgery, etc., but it is also a subsystem of the larger health care delivery system. The hospital system interacts with each of the internal subsystems plus

FAST FACTS in a NUTSHELL

- Nursing/staff development/patient teaching programs are subsystems of the larger educational institution or organization.
- Nursing/staff development/patient teaching programs are interdependent with the larger educational institution or organization.
- Internal/external factors affecting the larger educational institution or organization may also affect the nursing/staff development/patient teaching programs.

many external systems, such as regulatory agencies, community, third party payers, and others. Within a hospital system, the focus is on the arrangement of and the relations between the subsystems that connect them into the larger system.

Systems can acquire new properties through emergence, resulting in continual evolution. Changes in the health care delivery system from a focus on hospital care to outpatient care and an emphasis on wellness instead of illness are examples of this evolution. Systems can be chaos driven or purpose driven. For a system to function as a system, rather than a collection of parts, it must have ways of directing the behavior of the system (Trochim, Cabrera, Milstein, Gallagher, & Leischow, 2006). In order to be purpose driven, systems strive to maintain balance by effectively performing specific functions. Several of these functions include:

- The ability to adjust or adapt. Systems have the ability to cope with changes in the internal/external environments by acquiring necessary resources and through modification of self, the environment, or other systems to create a more welcoming state.
- The ability for goal attainment by setting priorities and using appropriate resources to obtain desired outcomes.
- The ability to integrate by organizing internally the activity of subsystems that make up the system. By constant readjustments, systems maintain motivation and deal with internal tensions.

Using systems theory to alter the way we think about educational programs can assist nurse educators in creating educational programs that perform effectively by adapting, achieving expected outcomes, and maintaining motivation to be purpose driven and not chaos driven. Educational programs continue to evolve over time as new information,

- All elements of a nursing program and nursing practice can use systems thinking to review, reorder, and reinforce to ensure that desired outcomes are achieved.
- Most educators are not accustomed to thinking in a systems fashion.

processes, or standards emerge. Using systems thinking as a framework, nurse educators will be able to analyze and/or describe any grouping of program elements and/or courses that work in concert to produce some result.

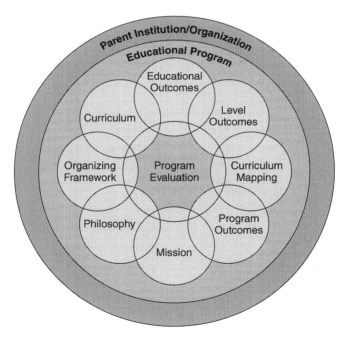

FIGURE 2.1   Systems thinking applied to a nursing program.

Figure 2.1 depicts the standard elements for a nursing or educational program. The elements that form a nursing/educational program system interact and are interdependent with all other elements. A nursing/educational program is also a subsystem within the larger system, whether higher education institution, organization with staff development requirements, or patient education needs.

While it is possible to use selected chapters to revise specific parts of a nursing program, remember that a program follows basic system theory principles and concepts. A nursing program system is an open system and individual program elements will change and evolve as changes occur in the parent institution, nursing practice standards, innovations in teaching and learning, etc. When making nursing program or course decisions, it is essential to constantly look forward and backward for desired and undesired effects, not only on the nursing/educational program but also on other subsystems within the larger educational institution, and the larger educational system itself.

3

Purposes and Development of a Mission Statement

INTRODUCTION

Every organization has a mission, a purpose, a reason for being. Organizations consider the development of a mission statement as a crucial factor in the creation of a business strategy. The mission statement is believed to promote a sense of shared expectations in employees and communicates to consumers why the organization exists. Meaningful mission statements can be viewed as a management tool critical to the success of an organization.

In this chapter, you will learn:

1. Why it is important to have a program mission statement.
2. The basic components of a mission statement.
3. How to develop a mission statement that is congruent with the parent organization.

PURPOSES OF A PROGRAM MISSION STATEMENT

A mission statement is a brief description of an organization's fundamental purpose both for those within the organization and for the public. It is a short written statement of an organization's business goals and philosophies and describes the organization's function, markets, and competitive advantages. A mission statement defines what an organization is, why it exists, and its reason for being. At a minimum, a mission statement should define the organization's primary customers, identify the products and services produced by the organization, and describe the geographical location in which the organization operates.

Within educational institutions, mission statements are declarations of a college's/university's rationale and purpose for existing; its responsibilities toward students and the community; and its vision of student, educator, and institutional excellence (Meacham, 2008). Nearly every college or university has a mission statement.

Definition of Key Terms

- **Mission statement** focuses on an organization's present state. The mission statement is an announcement of what the organization does today and why it exists.
- **Vision statement** focuses on an organization's future. A vision statement takes into account the current status of the organization, and is used to provide direction for the organization.
- **Brand** is the identity of a specific product, service, or business. It can take many forms, including a name, sign, symbol, color combination, or slogan. Stakeholders should be able to easily and quickly recognize a brand and immediately know what the organization strives to do. Many institutions of higher learning create brands to quickly catch the attention of students.

KEY POINTS

A good mission statement should accurately explain why your organization exists and what it hopes to achieve. The mission statement can be one sentence or a short paragraph, but must clearly communicate the organization/program's essential nature, its values, and its work to people within and outside the program.

purpose, business, values

=== *FAST FACTS in a NUTSHELL*

The typical elements of a program mission statement include:

- The purpose of the program
- The business of the program
- The values of the program

∅ task oriented

The mission statement is always bigger than a particular employment position; therefore, a specific position should not be part of the mission. The mission statement should not be task oriented. While there may be separate goal statements developed in order to accomplish the mission, the mission is a much broader statement.

Creating a program mission statement requires input from multiple stakeholders. The principal nursing program's stakeholders are students, educators, and consumers. Stakeholders for patient education courses are the recipients of care or their caregivers. Stakeholders for staff development courses are the employers and employees. Remember that an individual program is a subsystem of the larger organization; therefore, the program mission statement must be consistent with the organization's broader mission statement.

program mission statement must be consistent w/ org. mission statement!

===*FAST FACTS in a NUTSHELL*

The educational program's mission should complement and further the mission of the parent organization.

EXAMPLES OF A PROGRAM MISSION STATEMENT DEVELOPMENT

Before developing a nursing program mission statement, stakeholders must understand the mission of the organization/parent institution. The following example of the mission-building process improves understanding of the broader institutional mission and the role of the nursing program within that institution.

Organization/Parent Institution Mission Statement Worksheet (Table 3.1)

1. Insert the organization/parent institution's mission statement in Row 1 of the **Organization/Parent Institution Mission Statement Worksheet**.
2. Insert the questions to be asked about the organization/parent institution beliefs, business, and values found in the mission statement in Row 2, one question for each column.
3. Add sufficient space for responses below each question.
4. Distribute the **Organization/Parent Institution Mission Statement Worksheet** to stakeholders, asking each participant to answer the question in each column.
5. Collect and compile responses into a master list.
6. Distribute the master list and ask each stakeholder to review all responses on the master list in preparation for completing the **Nursing Program Mission Statement Worksheet**.

TABLE 3.1 Organization/Parent Institution Mission Statement Worksheet

(Insert the mission statement of the organization/parent institution.)

Based on the above mission statement, what is the purpose (why does it exist?) for the organization/ parent institution?	Based on the above mission statement, what is the business (what does it do?) of the organization/ parent institution?	Based on the above mission statement, what are the values (what does it believe?) of the organization/ parent institution?
Participants' responses: _____	Participants' responses: _____	Participants' responses: _____
_____	_____	_____
_____	_____	_____
_____	_____	_____
_____	_____	_____
_____	_____	_____
_____	_____	_____

═══════════*FAST FACTS in a NUTSHELL*

- Systems theory is evident within educational institutions where every program offered is a subsystem of the larger institution.
- Systems thinking can assist any school of nursing in the development a mission statement that contributes to and furthers the mission of the organization.

Nursing Program Mission Statement Worksheet (Table 3.2)

1. Distribute the **Nursing Program Mission Statement Worksheet** to multiple stakeholders for input on the three questions listed in Row 1. Be sure to provide a copy of the completed **Organization/Parent Institution Mission Statement Worksheet**.

2. Once input has been provided, compile the responses in a master list.
3. Distribute the master list and ask each stakeholder to review all responses on the master list and compose one sentence for each of the questions.
4. Compile a second master list containing all the one-sentence responses. It may be necessary to go back and forth before final acceptance occurs.

Once the final statements about program purpose, business, and values are accepted, compare the program statements to the statements from the organization/parent institution's mission statement. The program statements should further the organization/parent institution's mission by demonstrating congruency with and contributing to the accomplishment of the organization's mission statement. Table 3.3, **Comparison of Organization/Parent Institution Mission Statement and Nursing Program Mission Statement**, demonstrates one way to document consistency between organization/parent institution and program mission statements.

TABLE 3.2 Nursing Program Mission Statement Worksheet

(Insert the final nursing program mission statement. The mission statement should clearly and concisely express the program's purpose, business, and values.)

What is the purpose (why does the program exist?) for the nursing program?	What is the business (what does the program do?) of the nursing program?	What are the values (what does the program believe?) of the nursing program?
Participants' responses: _____	Participants' responses: _____	Participants' responses: _____
_____	_____	_____
_____	_____	_____
_____	_____	_____
_____	_____	_____

===*FAST FACTS in a NUTSHELL*

- Mission statements are dynamic and may need to be revised.
- Changes in internal factors, such as a change in the organization's mission statement and/or changes in external factors, such as changes in community needs, will require periodic review.

TABLE 3.3 Comparison of Organization/Parent Institution Mission Statement and Nursing Program Mission Statement

The Organization/Parent Institution Mission	The Nursing Program Mission
The organization/parent institution's purpose	The nursing program's purpose. Must clearly further the purpose of the parent institution
The organization/parent institution's business	The nursing program's business. Must clearly further the business of the parent institution
The organization/parent institution's values	The nursing program's values. Must clearly further the values of the parent institution

Subsequent chapters will add program elements to the **Comparison of Organization Mission Statement and Nursing Program Mission Statement** table (Table 3.3). Instructional mission statements are periodically reviewed and may be revised to reflect changes in purpose, business, and/or values. When this occurs, program mission statements must be revised to ensure congruency with the new institutional mission. Once the mission statement has been developed and congruency has been demonstrated, the next program element to be developed is the nursing program philosophy.

4

Purposes and Development of a Program Philosophy

INTRODUCTION

Once the program has a mission statement that aligns with the organization/parent institution's mission, it's time to develop a program philosophy. As with the mission statement, the program philosophy must align with the organization/parent institution's philosophy. If the organization/parent institution does not have a philosophy, then the program philosophy uses the organization/parent institution's mission statement. While the philosophy statement of the organization/parent institution will be broad in nature to cover all programs and services, the program philosophy is directed at the specific discipline. Developing a program philosophy statement requires reflection and insights about the discipline.

In this chapter, you will learn:

1. Why it is important to have a program philosophy.
2. The basic components of a program philosophy.
3. How to develop a program philosophy statement that is congruent with the parent organization and standards of nursing practice.

PURPOSES OF A PROGRAM PHILOSOPHY

The philosophy statement explains how the program mission is achieved and is used to make decisions about the program and the curriculum. The program philosophy presents a belief system that reflects what providers within the discipline believe about the discipline; the phenomena observed to exist in the discipline, the roles fulfilled, and the differences in roles with different levels of providers (Nursing Management, 2011). The program philosophy allows nursing programs to articulate beliefs about health, the recipients of care (individuals, families, groups, communities), the roles of the nurse, and the teaching/learning process.

==*FAST FACTS in a NUTSHELL*

A well-articulated philosophy will guide what is taught and how it will be taught.

Definition of Key Terms
- A **philosophy** is any system of beliefs, values, or tenets. It is also a personal outlook or viewpoint; a system of values by which one lives.
- A **program philosophy** is a set of ideas or beliefs relating to a particular field, discipline, or activity.

KEY POINTS

The typical elements of a nursing program philosophy include:

- Beliefs about the discipline, its phenomena, roles, relationships with other providers, relevant national standards, etc.

- Beliefs about health, illness, and wellness that include all dimensions of health—physiological, psychological, emotional, spiritual, and social health.
- Beliefs about the recipient of care (individuals, families, groups, communities) and their roles and responsibilities in maintaining or improving health.
- Beliefs about how learning occurs and how and what teaching needs to take place for learning to occur.

===*FAST FACTS in a NUTSHELL*

- The nursing program philosophy needs to be concise and to the point, but must have enough detail to guide program decisions.
- The length of a program philosophy will vary across programs, but the typical elements can be addressed in a page or two.

Input from nursing program educators is essential in developing a program philosophy. Educators teach what they believe to be true and the program philosophy statement must reflect the beliefs of the educator. Consensus building must occur. (include Educator beliefs)

===*FAST FACTS in a NUTSHELL*

- Similar to the mission statement, creating a program philosophy statement requires input from multiple stakeholders.
- The principal nursing program stakeholders are consumers, educators, and other health providers currently in practice.

Systems thinking is important when developing a nursing program philosophy statement. An individual program is a subset of the bigger organization; therefore, the nursing program philosophy statement must be consistent with the organization's philosophy statement. If the organization does not have a philosophy statement, the mission statement of the organization is used.

FAST FACTS in a NUTSHELL

The nursing program's philosophy should complement the philosophy/mission statement of the parent organization.

EXAMPLE OF NURSING PROGRAM PHILOSOPHY DEVELOPMENT

Before developing a nursing program philosophy, educators and current members of the discipline must understand the mission and philosophy of the organization/parent institution. The following example will improve understanding of the broader mission and philosophy of the organization/parent institution and how the nursing program is congruent within this broader context.

Organization/Parent Institution Philosophy Statement Worksheet (Table 4.1)

1. Distribute the **Philosophy Statement Worksheet** to educators and current providers of the discipline.
2. Based on the philosophy statement for the organization/parent institution, request participants to identify the

---

TABLE 4.1 Organization/Parent Institution Philosophy Statement Worksheet

(Insert the organization/parent institution's philosophy statement. If the organization/parent institution does not have a philosophy statement, use the mission statement.)

Ideas of the organization/parent institution	**Beliefs** of the organization/parent institution	**Values** of the organization/parent institution
————————	————————	————————
————————	————————	————————
————————	————————	————————
————————	————————	————————

---

    ideas, beliefs, and values the organization/parent institution uses to implement its philosophy. Participants cannot change the organization/parent institution philosophy.

3. Compile the participants' responses and share the master list with all.

═══════════════════════*FAST FACTS in a NUTSHELL*

When the organization does not have a separate philosophy statement, the mission statement is used to demonstrate congruency between the organization and the nursing program.

Nursing Program Philosophy Statement Worksheet (Table 4.2)

1. Distribute the **Nursing Program Philosophy Statement Worksheet** to program educators and providers currently in practice, requesting input.

2. Once input has been provided, compile responses in a master list.
3. Distribute the master list and ask each participant to condense the responses to a concise statement for each of the areas.
4. Compile a master list again and compare responses to the statements from the organization/parent institution's philosophy (mission) statement. It may be necessary to go back and forth until the nursing program statements can be viewed as furthering the organization/parent institution's philosophy (mission).

TABLE 4.2 Nursing Program Philosophy Statement Worksheet

Philosophy Statement Guidelines	Nursing Program Philosophy
Write a concise statement about the beliefs that reflect what providers within the discipline believe about the discipline; the phenomena observed to exist in the discipline, the roles fulfilled, and the differences in roles with different levels of providers. Include applicable national standards.	_____ _____ _____ _____ _____ _____ _____ _____
Write a concise statement about what health encompasses. Include applicable national standards.	_____ _____ _____
Write a concise statement about the recipients of care (individuals, families, groups, communities). What are their main characteristics, roles, and responsibilities related to health? Include applicable national standards.	_____ _____ _____ _____ _____ _____
Write a concise statement about the teaching/learning process. How do individuals, families, groups, and communities learn, and what teaching processes will accomplish learning? Include applicable national standards.	_____ _____ _____ _____ _____ _____

The philosophy statement should not be a list of tasks. There may be separate goal statements developed in order to accomplish the philosophy. Goal statements must be congruent with the parent institution and clarify what the nursing program intends to accomplish.

Using the final product from the Table 4.1, **Organization/ Parent Institution Philosophy Statement Worksheet**, and Table 4.2, **Nursing Program Philosophy Statement Worksheet**, combine into one table to demonstrate congruency (Table 4.3).

TABLE 4.3 Comparison of Organization/Parent Institution Philosophy (Mission) Statement and Nursing Program Mission and Philosophy Statement

Organization/Parent Institution Mission/ Philosophy	Nursing Program Mission	Nursing Program Philosophy
The organization/ parent institution's mission and philosophy (purpose, beliefs, values)	The nursing program's mission (purpose, beliefs, values)	The nursing program's philosophy is aligned with the mission/philosophy of the organization/ parent institution as evidenced by: (insert statements from the program philosophy that are consistent with the ideas of the organization/parent institution)
(Developed in Chapter 3 example)	*(Developed in Chapter 3 example)*	

The completion of the worksheets in Tables 4.1 and 4.2 should assist in the development of a meaningful nursing program philosophy statement that is congruent with the philosophy (or mission) statement of the organization/ parent institution. Like mission statements, philosophy statements are dynamic and need periodic review depending on changes in internal or external factors. Subsequent chapters will continue to add program elements to the **Comparison of Organization and Nursing Program** table (Table 4.3). The next program element to be developed is the nursing program organizing framework.

5

Purposes and Selection of an Organizing Framework

(re. conceptual & curriculum frameworks)

INTRODUCTION

The literature may refer to organizing frameworks as conceptual frameworks, curriculum frameworks, or another term. Regardless of the label, organizing frameworks are a <u>collection of concepts that form a construct in which each concept plays an integral role</u>. Once the program has a mission statement that aligns with the organization's mission and a program philosophy, it's time to construct an organizing framework. The organizing framework must align with the nursing program philosophy. It is from the nursing program philosophy the major concepts are identified and defined. While some of the major concepts may reflect the broad student attributes of the organization, such as critical thinking, communication, and computer literacy, they also include concepts specific to the discipline of nursing, such as health, professional skills, and standards of practice. Constructing an organizing framework requires reflection and insight about the discipline.

• align w/ philosophy

In this chapter, you will learn:

1. Why it is important to have an organizing framework.
2. The basic components of an organizing framework.
3. How to develop an organizing framework that is congruent with the nursing program philosophy and guides curriculum development.

PURPOSES OF AN ORGANIZING FRAMEWORK

The general purpose of an organizing framework is to create a structure for building the nursing program's curriculum. The framework isolates the concepts identified in the nursing program philosophy and relates them to standards of practice and employer and consumer expectations. The organizing framework acts as the building blocks or foundation for the curriculum. It provides a frame of reference for members of a discipline to guide their thinking, observations, and interpretations.

Definition of Key Terms
- A **concept** is an idea of something formed by mentally combining all its characteristics.
- A **construct** is the creation of an idea, image, or theory by systematically arranging a number of simple or complex elements.
- An **organizing framework** is a group of concepts that are broadly defined and systematically organized to provide a focus, a rationale, and a tool for the integration and interpretation of information (Jabareen, 2009). Organizing frameworks also provide a foundation and organization for the educational plan in nursing programs. Frameworks provide a basis for thinking about what we do and about what it means, influenced by the ideas and research of others.

KEY POINTS

An organizing framework establishes the shared vision for the educational program's efforts in preparing nurses, updating current health care providers, or preparing consumers to care for themselves. It provides direction for programs, courses, teaching, student performance, scholarship, service, and program accountability. The organizing framework is knowledge-based, articulated, shared, coherent, consistent with the program and institutional missions, and continuously evaluated. It provides the base that describes the program's intellectual philosophy.

An organizing framework helps explain why the curriculum has been set up in a particular way. It also helps to understand and use the ideas of others who have done similar things.

FAST FACTS in a NUTSHELL

An organizing framework is used like a travel map. The framework helps educators decide and explain the route to be taken: why certain methods are used to reach a certain point and why others are not used.

"threads" → concepts

In the past, "threads" was the common term used to refer to the identified curriculum organizing themes (concepts). Threads were designated as being either vertical or horizontal. Vertical threads represented the themes (concepts) that were introduced at a lower level and grew or became more complex as learners advanced in the program. An example of a vertical thread would be the roles of the nurse. Most nursing programs expand role functions as the learner progresses through the program; the nursing roles become more complex.

Horizontal threads represent themes (concepts) that are present throughout all courses. Health would be an example of a horizontal thread, since nursing programs often address some aspect of health in all courses.

Some educators use the terms "progressive" and "pervasive" to differentiate between vertical and horizontal. Progressive threads serve the same purpose as vertical threads, moving from simple to complex. Likewise, pervasive and horizontal threads are the same; present in every course. *pervasive vs. progressive*

Identification of threads assists in organizing the curriculum. It creates a curricular foundation by weaving the vertical and horizontal threads into a strong fabric.

Identifying the themes (concepts) is more important than labeling them as vertical or horizontal. Designating themes (concepts) as vertical or horizontal at times can seem arbitrary. Using the examples above:

- The role of provider could be labeled horizontal because the provider role is presented in all courses.
- Health could move in complexity throughout the program from wellness to acute illness to chronic illness to comorbidity.

===*FAST FACTS in a NUTSHELL*

- Themes come directly from the nursing program philosophy and are referred to as concepts.
- The concepts are used as the foundation for the curriculum and help organize and implement the program of study.
- Major concepts may have a number of characteristics, which can be designated as subconcepts.

In Chapter 4, the typical elements for a program philosophy were identified (beliefs about nursing, health, recipient of care, and learning) and can be the starting point for identifying additional concepts. Examples of some additional concepts include safety, communication, cultural diversity, collaboration, respect for others, and professional behavior.

Once the organizing concepts have been identified, they must be defined. The definitions will clearly explain to the learner, other educators, employers, and consumers what the concepts mean. Typically, the definitions reflect what the educators believe, the industry standards, and employer and consumer expectations. Outside references are often used to strengthen the definitions.

Many organizations have core outcomes for all graduates regardless of program of study. These outcomes, often referred to as student attributes or abilities, may or may not be specific to the nursing program's philosophy but should be included as concepts within the organizing framework. Examples of organization-wide outcomes include critical thinking, computer literacy, communication (written and verbal), and mathematical computation. In order to demonstrate congruency with the organization's mission, the broader core outcomes must be included in the organizing concepts for the nursing program.

===*FAST FACTS in a NUTSHELL*

The organizing framework must clearly demonstrate a flow from the nursing program mission and philosophy. If the concepts have been taken directly from the nursing program philosophy, this flow will be evident.

EXAMPLES OF ORGANIZING FRAMEWORK DEVELOPMENT

Before developing a nursing program organizing framework, educators must understand and agree with the nursing program's philosophy statement. In addition, the educators must be familiar with the core outcomes for all graduates as defined by the organization/parent institution. The concepts for the organizing framework come directly from the nursing program's philosophy and the organization/parent institution identifies and defines the core outcomes for all graduates. The following worksheets will assist in identifying the concepts relating to the core outcomes and the critical concepts contained in the nursing program's philosophy.

Organization/Parent Institution Core Outcomes (Concepts) Worksheet (Table 5.1)

Many institutions develop general core outcomes all learners must achieve by graduation. The core student outcomes are an integral component of the organizing framework for all degree programs, including nursing. Core outcomes will vary between institutions, but critical thinking, communication, and mathematical computation are frequent.

Table 5.1 will assist educators in developing nursing program–specific definitions for the core outcomes (concepts) while maintaining congruency with the definitions of the organization/parent institution.

1. Create a three-column table. In the first column (left column), list the organization/parent institution's core outcomes for all graduates as a concept.
2. In the second column (middle column), place the organization/parent institution's definition of the concept.
3. The third column is left blank for now.
4. Distribute the **Organization/Parent Institution Core Outcomes (Concepts) Worksheet** to educators and request they develop a nursing program definition for each core outcome (concept). Nursing definitions must be consistent with the nursing program philosophy.

5. Participants cannot change items in the first two columns.
6. Once educators have completed their definitions, collect and compile responses from the third column and share the master list with all participants.
7. The educators should discuss the compiled definitions, formulating one definition that aligns with the general definition of the organization/parent institution and the nursing program's philosophy.

TABLE 5.1 Organization/Parent Institution Core Outcomes (Concepts) Worksheet

Organization/ Parent Institution Core Outcomes (Concepts)	Organization/ Institution Definition of Core Outcomes	Nursing Program Definition	Nursing Program Philosophy
Critical thinking (example)	How does the organization/ institution define "critical thinking"?	How does the nursing program define "critical thinking"?	Which nursing philosophy statement(s) best support the definition of "critical thinking"?
Communication (example)	How does the organization/ institution define "communication"?	How does the nursing program define "communication"?	Which nursing philosophy statement(s) best support the definition of "communication"?
Mathematical computation	How does the organization/ institution define "mathematical computation"?	How does the nursing program define "mathematical computation"?	Which nursing philosophy statement(s) best support the definition of "mathematical computation"?

Nursing Program Organizing Concepts
Worksheet (Table 5.2)

Once the educators have agreed on the nursing program definitions for the broader organization/institution core outcomes
(concepts), it's time to identify the nursing program concepts.
The nursing program concepts should be directly related to and
taken from the nursing program philosophy. The most common and frequently used major concepts are nursing, patient
(recipient of care), health, environment, and teaching/learning.

1. Create a three-column table and label one column for the
   nursing concept, one column for subconcepts, and the last
   for definitions of the major concepts.
2. Distribute the **Nursing Program Organizing Concepts
   Worksheet** to all educators, requesting that each educator
   list the nursing program concepts contained in the program philosophy statement.
3. In the first column (left column), list each major concept
   identified in the program philosophy. In the second column, list any subconcepts for the major concepts. At this
   point, do nothing with the last column.
4. Collect and compile the educator responses and share the
   master list with all participants.
5. The educators should discuss the list of nursing program
   organizing concepts, narrowing it down to the major concepts to be used in organizing the curriculum. Educators
   should closely examine the master list of nursing program
   concepts carefully. Save the list of subconcepts since they
   will be used when mapping the curriculum.
6. If concepts are identified at this time that are not in the
   nursing program philosophy, it may be necessary to return to the philosophy for revision.
7. Finalize the list of nursing program concepts and place in
   a new table. Make sure concepts required by approval or
   accrediting agencies have been included.

TABLE 5.2 Program Organizing Concepts and Definitions

Major Program Concepts	Subconcepts	Definitions of Major Program Concepts
Person (recipient of care)	What subconcepts relate to "person"?	How does the nursing philosophy define "person"?
Environment	What subconcepts relate to "environment"?	How does the nursing philosophy define "environment"?
Nursing (nursing practice, standards, and roles)	What subconcepts relate to "nursing"?	How does the nursing philosophy define "nursing"?
Health	What subconcepts relate to "health"?	How does the nursing philosophy define "health"?
Teaching/learning	What subconcepts relate to "teaching/learning"?	How does the nursing philosophy define "teaching/learning"?

8. Distribute the final list of program concepts to all educators, requesting they develop a definition for each nursing program concept.
9. Collect and compile the educator definitions and share the master list with all participants.
10. The educators should discuss the compiled definitions, formulating one definition that aligns with the program philosophy and the organization/institution core outcomes (concepts).

Table 5.3 demonstrates how to align the concepts from a specific program with the broader concepts of the organization. Further refinement of the nursing definitions would be necessary, but the example demonstrates that the core outcomes (concepts) can easily be incorporated into the nursing program concepts.

FAST FACTS in a NUTSHELL

The core outcomes (concepts) of the organization do not have to be addressed separately from the nursing program concepts.

TABLE 5.3 Alignment of Nursing Program/Institution Concepts/Definitions With Program Philosophy

Parent Institution Core Outcomes	Nursing Program's Philosophy	Nursing Program Major Concepts	Nursing Program Definitions for Core Outcomes and Major Concepts
Examples: Critical thinking	Statements from the nursing program philosophy that support the major organizing concept.		How does the nursing philosophy define "critical thinking"?
Communication	Statements from the nursing program philosophy that support the major organizing concept.		How does the nursing philosophy define "communication"?
Mathematical computation	Statements from the nursing program philosophy that support the major organizing concept.		How does the nursing philosophy define "mathematical computation"?

(continued)

TABLE 5.3 Alignment of Nursing Program/Institution Concepts/Definitions With Program Philosophy (*continued*)

Parent Institution Core Outcomes	Nursing Program's Philosophy	Nursing Program Major Concepts	Nursing Program Definitions for Core Outcomes and Major Concepts
	Statements from the nursing program philosophy that support the major organizing concept.	Nursing	How does the nursing philosophy define "nursing"?
	Statements from the nursing program philosophy that support the major organizing concept.	Person (recipient of care)	How does the nursing philosophy define "person"?
	Statements from the nursing program philosophy that support the major organizing concept.	Environment	How does the nursing philosophy define "environment"?
	Statements from the nursing program philosophy that support the major organizing concept.	Health	How does the nursing philosophy define "health"?

(continued)

TABLE 5.3 Alignment of Nursing Program/Institution Concepts/Definitions With Program Philosophy (continued)

Parent Institution Core Outcomes	Nursing Program's Philosophy	Nursing Program Major Concepts	Nursing Program Definitions for Core Outcomes and Major Concepts
	Statements from the nursing program philosophy that support the major organizing concept.	Teaching and learning	How does the nursing philosophy define "teaching and learning"?

The above examples should assist in the development of an organizing framework that is congruent with the nursing program philosophy and the core outcomes of the organization. As with the mission and philosophy statements, organizing frameworks are dynamic and may need to be adjusted depending on internal and/or external factors (e.g., practice standards, approval/accrediting agency requirements, employer expectations); therefore, periodic review is necessary. Once the organizing framework has been developed, it's time to develop the program's educational outcomes.

Educational and Level Outcomes

6

Purposes and Examples
of Educational Outcomes

*(performance outcomes,
competency outcomes
or objectives)*

INTRODUCTION

*Educational outcomes delineate what you want your
learners to know and be able to do at the completion of
the nursing program. The term, educational outcomes, is
used to distinguish between nursing program outcomes
and those course outcomes resulting from the teaching/
learning process. Educational outcomes are referred to
using a variety of terms, such as, performance outcomes,
competency outcomes, or objectives. So far, the nursing
program mission, philosophy statement, and the organizing framework have been developed. The development of
educational outcomes will build on this previous work.*

In this chapter, you will learn:

1. Why it is important to have well-articulated educational outcomes
   for the nursing program.
2. How to develop educational outcomes that are congruent with the
   nursing program philosophy and organizing framework.

PURPOSES OF EDUCATIONAL OUTCOMES

- The purpose of educational outcomes is to identify the performance level required of learners at completion of the educational experience, such as the nursing program (Wittmann-Price & Fasolka, 2010). Educational outcomes articulate and communicate what graduates must know and be able to do as they exit the nursing program.
- Achievement of educational outcomes focuses on results, not inputs and processes.

===*FAST FACTS in a NUTSHELL*

The achievement of educational outcomes is the major focus, not the textbooks or instructional style used. The best textbooks and instructional methods do not guarantee achievement of educational outcomes. Textbooks and instructional methods are considered inputs and processes to assist in achieving educational outcomes.

objective = goal
outcome = consequence

Definition of Key Terms

- An **outcome** is defined as an end result; a consequence.
- An **objective** is defined as something that one's efforts or actions are intended to attain or accomplish; something worked toward or strived for; a purpose; a goal.
- An **educational, performance, or competency outcome** is defined as the observable behaviors and actions that explain how the job is to be done; it communicates expectations.

KEY POINTS

Educational outcomes reflect the knowledge, actions, beliefs, and values of the discipline and expectations of employers and consumers. They must flow from the nursing program philosophy and organizing framework.

The educational outcome should answer the question: "What will the participant be able to do as a result of the nursing program educational experience?" Educational outcomes must clearly delineate the performance or competencies expected by the learner at the completion of the educational experience and should aim to describe a behavior that is measurable.

════════════════════════════*FAST FACTS in a NUTSHELL*

> Educational outcomes, written in clear, demonstrable language, are used to guide learner assessment, direct curriculum development, and evaluate effectiveness of instruction.

Educational outcomes are the criteria used to select materials, outline content, develop instructional procedures, and prepare tests and examinations. No valid assessment can be developed without a clear delineation of the educational outcome upon which the assessment is based. It is important to keep your eye on the outcomes for a nursing program, not on the inputs or processes.

Educational outcomes must be learner rather than educator based. Keep in mind the purpose of education is to bring about measurable changes in the learners' patterns of behavior, not to have the educator perform certain activities.

The actual number of educational outcomes will vary from nursing program to nursing program. The number of

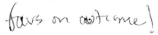

educational outcomes must be reasonable. Too many educational outcomes may make it difficult for educators to measure and learners to demonstrate competency. Too few educational outcomes may not accurately delineate discipline standards and employer/consumer expectations. Eight to twelve educational outcomes would be reasonable.

Accrediting organizations require nursing programs to have stated outcomes that are based on practice standards and the identified needs of the client population.

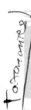

=========================*FAST FACTS in a NUTSHELL*

Educational taxonomies (cognitive, affective, psychomotor) are useful guides to understanding and writing educational outcomes.

EXAMPLES OF DEVELOPING EDUCATIONAL OUTCOMES

Before developing educational outcomes, educators must understand and agree with the nursing program organizing framework. The concepts for the organizing framework and the organization/parent institution are the building blocks for the educational outcomes. The following example will assist educators in using the core outcomes for all graduates as defined by the organization/parent institution, and the nursing program organizing framework concepts to develop the nursing program educational outcomes.

Nursing Program Educational Outcomes Example

This example will assist educators in developing educational outcomes congruent with the nursing program mission/philosophy and organizing framework while maintaining congruency with the organization/parent institution purpose.

The simplest way to approach the task of developing educational outcomes is to use the major organizing concepts developed in a previous chapter.

1. Create a two-column table with sufficient rows to list all organizing concepts, organizational/institutional as well as nursing program. If there are more than twelve concepts, closer examination may identify some that can be defined as subconcepts, thus shortening the list.

2. Distribute the **Nursing Program Educational Outcomes Worksheet** to all educators, requesting that each educator develop, in the second column, an educational outcome for each concept. The educational outcome must include a performance expectation and a content area. The performance expectation and content area should directly relate to the organizing framework concept. The educational outcome should clearly communicate to the learner what they must demonstrate to meet the end-of-program expectations.

3. Collect and compile all educator-developed educational outcomes and share the master worksheet with all participants.

4. The educators should discuss all proposed educational outcomes on the master worksheet and agree on performance expectations, content, and wording.

5. If educational outcomes are identified at this time that are not in the nursing program organizing framework, it may be necessary to return to all previous nursing program documents for inclusion of additional concepts and necessary revisions.

6. Finalize the list of educational outcomes and place in a new table.

Table 6.1 provides an example of how to align the organizing concepts with the educational outcomes.

TABLE 6.1 Educational Outcomes Example

Organizing Concepts	Nursing Program Educational Outcome
Person	End-of-program performance and knowledge expectation for the concept of "person"
Environment	End-of-program performance and knowledge expectation for the concept of "environment"
Nursing	End-of-program performance and knowledge expectation for the concept of "nursing"
Health	End-of-program performance and knowledge expectation for the concept of "health"
Teaching/learning	End-of-program performance and knowledge expectation for the concept of "teaching/learning"
Communication	End-of-program performance and knowledge expectation for the concept of "communication"
Critical thinking	End-of-program performance and knowledge expectation for the concept of "critical thinking"
Mathematical computation	End-of-program performance and knowledge expectation for the concept of "mathematical computation"

Table 6.2 provides an example of educational outcomes that are congruent with the nursing program mission/philosophy and organizing framework. The assumption is made that if the program's educational outcomes are congruent with the program mission/philosophy and organizing framework, then congruency with the organization mission/philosophy has been maintained.

TABLE 6.2 Comparison of Nursing Program Philosophy Statement, Organizing Framework, and Educational Outcomes

Nursing Program Philosophy	Nursing Program Organizing Framework	Nursing Program Educational Outcomes
Show that the nursing program philosophy is aligned with the mission/philosophy of the organization/parent institution by inserting statements from the nursing program philosophy that demonstrate consistency.	Show that the nursing program organizing framework is aligned with the nursing program philosophy and the institutional core concepts by inserting concepts with definitions that demonstrate consistency.	Show that the nursing program educational outcomes are aligned with the nursing program philosophy, organizing framework, and the core concepts of the parent institution by inserting the educational outcomes that demonstrate consistency.

The examples should assist educators in the development of meaningful nursing program educational outcomes that are congruent with the mission/philosophy statements and organizing framework of the nursing program, practice standards, and the organization. Like the previous program elements, educational outcomes are dynamic and may need to be adjusted depending on changes in internal factors (e.g., changes in mission/philosophy statements with either the organization or nursing program, changes in the organizing framework) and external factors (e.g., practice standards, approval/accrediting standards, employer expectations); therefore, educational outcomes require periodic review. Once the educational outcomes have been developed, it's time to level the educational outcomes.

7

Purposes and Examples
of Level Outcomes

INTRODUCTION

Some programs have multiple nursing levels, such as practical nurse, associate degree nurse, or baccalaureate degree nurse. Nursing programs with multiple levels find it helpful to use educational outcomes as a way to better define the performance expectations necessary to progress from one program to the next. Programs requiring multiple semesters for completion find it helpful to use the educational outcomes as a way to better define the performance expectations necessary to progress from semester to semester. Leveling the educational outcomes by program level or by end-of-semester expectations guides educators so educational experiences are at an appropriate level for the learner and demonstrate progression.

In this chapter, you will learn:

1. Why it is important to level the expected outcomes for a nursing program.
2. How to level outcomes in a nursing program to pace and sequence learning and promote the achievement of expected outcomes.

progresses from simple to complex

PURPOSES OF LEVEL OUTCOMES

Leveling of program outcomes typically begins with the program's educational outcomes. Since level outcomes are derived from the educational outcomes, leveling allows learners to progress from simpler expectations to more complex expectations (Duignan, 2009). Leveling the educational outcomes allows educators to design a curriculum that progresses from simple to complex expectations over a specified time period, such as a semester, an academic year, or between different types of programs (practical, associate degree, baccalaureate). Each level permits learners and educators to build on previous knowledge, attitudes, and skills.

Definition of Key Terms
- **Level outcomes** are statements that specify what learners will know or be able to do as a result of a learning unit.
- **Level outcomes** are statements that describe a desired condition.

KEY POINTS

Level outcomes should flow from and directly link to the educational outcomes. The number of levels is a decision made by the nursing program faculty. There can be as many levels as there are semesters in the program or as few as levels between programs.

The number of levels is an educator/program decision. Many times nursing programs require more than one course within a given semester. Leveling takes into consideration all courses within a given semester and assists educators in designing learning experiences directed at achieving the desired level of learning so learners will be prepared for subsequent semesters.

FAST FACTS in a NUTSHELL

Leveling each semester helps focus the learner on the performance expectations for that semester and for progression to the next semester.

Developing level outcomes is similar to developing course outcomes. When writing level outcomes:

- Focus on the learner's behavior that is to be changed (cognitive, affective, psychomotor).
- Identify specifically what should be learned at each level.
- Communicate to learners exactly what is expected and to be accomplished at the completion of the specified level.

Level outcomes should contain the following three elements:

- A specified action that is observable.
- A specified action that is performed by the learner.
- The specified action performed by the learner must be measurable.

The learner's performance must be observable and measurable. Similar to course outcomes, the verb chosen for each outcome statement should be an action verb that results in purposeful behavior that can be observed and measured. The ultimate test when writing a level outcome is whether the action taken by the learner can be assessed. If the level outcome cannot be assessed, the level outcome probably needs revision.

FAST FACTS in a NUTSHELL

Level outcomes should serve as guidelines for content, instruction, and evaluation at the specified level.

EXAMPLES OF LEVEL OUTCOME DEVELOPMENT

Before developing nursing program level outcomes, educators must understand and agree with the nursing program educational outcomes. The nursing program educational outcomes should clearly present the program performance expectations as learners exit the program. Leveling outcomes will break up the end-of-program expectations into smaller, incremental steps.

Nursing Program Level Outcomes Worksheet

This exercise will assist educators in developing nursing program level outcomes congruent with the nursing program mission/philosophy statements, organizing framework, and educational outcomes.

1. Create a simple table with a column for the number of levels desired. There should be sufficient rows to list all nursing program educational outcomes.
2. Place each nursing program educational outcome, developed in a previous chapter, in the far right-hand column, one outcome per row.
3. Distribute the **Nursing Program Level Outcomes Worksheet** to all educators. Request each educator develop a corresponding outcome, aligned with each nursing program educational outcome, for each level. The first level outcome will have the lowest performance/knowledge expectations. Each subsequent level outcome should build on the previous level expectations. The goal is to incrementally bring the learner to the end-of-program expectations, such as the educational outcomes. Like the nursing program educational outcomes, the nursing program level outcomes must include a performance expectation and a content area. The performance and content expectations should be directly related to the organizing framework concepts.
4. Collect and compile all educator-developed level outcomes and share the master worksheet with all participants.

5. The educators should discuss all proposed level outcomes on the master worksheet and agree on performance expectations, content, and wording across all levels.
6. There may be disagreement about leveling some performance expectations. Safety is an example. Some may argue that safe practice cannot be leveled. They will question how a learner can be a little safe in the first level and a little safer in subsequent levels. It is permissible not to level such outcomes as safe practice.
7. Finalize the list of nursing program level outcomes and place in a new table. The table should demonstrate the flow, left to right, of how the level outcomes build on previous outcomes to eventually achieve the educational outcomes for the program.

Table 7.1 is an example of leveling using two levels. The educational outcomes developed in a previous chapter should be used to develop the levels. Level outcomes must be congruent with the nursing program mission/philosophy statements, organizing framework, and educational outcomes. Additional levels might be required to show articulation from one program to the next, such as practical, associate degree, and/or baccalaureate.

TABLE 7.1 Example of Two Outcome Levels

Organizing Concept	Level 1	Level 2	Educational Outcome
Communication (core concept)	Beginning performance and knowledge expectation for the concept of "communication."	When combined with Level 1 outcome, should accomplish the educational outcome for "communication."	End-of-program performance and knowledge expectation for the concept of "communication."
Mathematical computation (core concept)	Beginning performance and knowledge expectation for the concept of "mathematical computation."	When combined with Level 1 outcome, should accomplish the educational outcome for "mathematical computation."	End-of-program performance and knowledge expectation for the concept of "mathematical computation."
Critical thinking (core concept)	Beginning performance and knowledge expectation for the concept of "critical thinking."	When combined with Level 1 outcome, should accomplish the educational outcome for "critical thinking."	End-of-program performance and knowledge expectation for the concept of "critical thinking."
Nursing (program concept)	Beginning performance and knowledge expectation for the concept of "nursing."	When combined with Level 1 outcome, should accomplish the educational outcome for "nursing."	End-of-program performance and knowledge expectation for the concept of "nursing."

Person (program concept)	Beginning performance and knowledge expectation for the concept of "person."	When combined with Level 1 outcome, should accomplish the educational outcome for "person."	End-of-program performance and knowledge expectation for the concept of "person."
Health (program concept)	Beginning performance and knowledge expectation for the concept of "health."	When combined with Level 1 outcome, should accomplish the educational outcome for "health."	End-of-program performance and knowledge expectation for the concept of "health."
Environment (program concept)	Beginning performance and knowledge expectation for the concept of "environment."	When combined with Level 1 outcome, should accomplish the educational outcome for "environment."	End-of-program performance and knowledge expectation for the concept of "environment."
Teaching/learning (program concept)	Beginning performance and knowledge expectation for the concept of "teaching/learning."	When combined with Level 1 outcome, should accomplish the educational outcome for "teaching/learning."	End-of-program performance and knowledge expectation for the concept of "teaching/learning."

The example should guide educators in the development of meaningful nursing program level outcomes that are congruent with previous structural elements of the nursing program as well as established practice standards. Like the mission/philosophy statements, organizing framework, and educational outcomes, level outcomes are dynamic and may need to be adjusted depending on changes in internal factors (e.g., changes in mission/philosophy statements with either the organization/parent institution or program, changes in the organizing framework or the educational outcomes) and external factors (e.g., changes in practice standards, approval/accrediting standards, employer expectations); therefore, level outcomes require periodic review. Once the level outcomes have been developed, it is time to examine the curriculum mapping process.

8

Purposes and Examples
of Curricular Mapping

INTRODUCTION

As you have worked through the various elements of a nursing program, you should have noticed the relationship, interaction and interdependence, between all elements. If one element is changed, all elements must be examined to see if the change affects them. If it does, then revisions must be made to align with any and all changes. Mapping of the concepts and subconcepts from the organizing framework and weaving them into the identified levels will show progression toward achieving the nursing program educational outcomes. Nursing programs with multiple levels find it helpful to use the educational outcomes as a way to better define the performance expectations necessary to progress from one program to the next. Mapping continues to build on previous program elements and helps develop and implement the curriculum; it determines what concepts will be introduced, when they will be introduced, and how each semester is to build on the previous semester's level expectations. Mapping the curriculum will guide educators with course development so educational experiences are at an appropriate level and demonstrate progression, reduce duplication, and minimize gaps.

In this chapter, you will learn:

1. Why it is important to map the curriculum for a nursing program.
2. How to map the nursing program curriculum in order to promote learning and achieve the educational outcomes of the program.

PURPOSES OF CURRICULAR MAPPING

- The purpose of a curriculum map is to document the relationship between every component of the curriculum (Harden, 2001). Mapping is used to analyze, plan, and communicate the curriculum. A curriculum map allows educators to review the curriculum for unnecessary redundancies, inconsistencies, misalignments, weaknesses, and gaps.
- Curriculum mapping documents the relationships between the required components of the curriculum and the intended learner outcomes.
- Mapping gives a broad picture of the taught curriculum and is a powerful tool for managing the curriculum.

Definition of Key Terms
- **Curriculum mapping** is a process for collecting and recording curriculum-related data that identifies core skills and content taught, instructional processes, and assessments used for each concept area and program level. The completed curriculum map becomes a tool that assists educators to track what has been taught and plan for what will be taught.

KEY POINTS

Curriculum mapping clearly demonstrates systems theory principles and concepts. When viewed from a systems perspective, the foundational documents (program mission, philosophy, organizing framework, educational outcomes, and level outcomes) act as subsystems within the program system.

━━━━━━━━━━━━━━━━━━━━━━━*FAST FACTS in a NUTSHELL*

Mapping provides a visual depiction of how the subsystems interact and interrelate and how they are interdependent.

Expanding the system to the organization/parent institution level, curriculum mapping also helps identify opportunities for integration of other disciplines (e.g., anatomy, physiology, English composition, etc.) (Cuevas, Matveev, & Miller, 2010).

━━━━━━━━━━━━━━━━━━━━━━━*FAST FACTS in a NUTSHELL*

• Curriculum maps should include how general education courses and the broader learner attributes for all graduates link to discipline-specific material.

Curriculum mapping can demonstrate congruency between the intended, delivered, and received curricula. It answers the question, "Is the real curriculum being taught?" Curriculum mapping also helps to identify potential deficiencies in the curriculum and aids in planning assessment activities and developing different models to guide the assessment process for approval/accrediting agencies.

At the program level, curriculum mapping provides a broad picture of how the program intends to achieve its educational outcomes. Using the level outcomes to divide the learning competencies over a specified period of time, it allows for incremental introduction and achievement of knowledge and skills necessary to accomplish the educational outcomes.

===*FAST FACTS in a NUTSHELL*

Curriculum mapping identifies what learners have learned, allowing educators to focus on building on previous knowledge.

Mapping the curriculum using concept maps is an effective way to explain subject matter understanding through a visual approach. The basic structure of major concepts and the visual depiction of the relationships among them can enhance understanding of a specific discipline for both educators and learners.

Curriculum mapping has many benefits.

- Curriculum mapping, using the concepts identified in the organizing framework and identifying the dominant relationships among the concepts, further clarifies what learning activities are needed to assist learners in demonstrating achievement of stated outcomes.
- In addition to mapping the organizing concepts, curriculum mapping includes the mapping of subconcepts, content, and assessments for all courses, whether preexisting or new.
- Curriculum mapping can be a useful process for quality assurance when assessments are designed to measure achievement of the level/educational outcomes.
- Curriculum mapping can present evidence of what learners actually learned in their courses rather than assumptions of what was learned based on content presented.
- Curriculum mapping can identify gaps or unnecessary redundancies in course learning activities.
- Curriculum mapping can demonstrate that learning activities are current, relevant, and taught at the appropriate level, allowing learners to achieve the appropriate educational outcomes level.

- Curriculum mapping can demonstrate when a course is taught, appropriateness of course prerequisites, and whether the course is offered in the best semester or professional year of the program.
- Curriculum mapping can demonstrate what measures are used to determine if learners achieved the desired learning outcomes (course, level, and program), how learners are assessed, and if the assessments align with course and program outcomes.

FAST FACTS in a NUTSHELL

Curriculum mapping at the course level can demonstrate:

- The instructional methods used
- The balance between acquiring and applying knowledge
- The learning resources and opportunities available
- The level of integration into the curriculum
- The comprehensiveness of the syllabus
- The appropriateness of the learner workload

Narrowing curriculum mapping to the course level allows educators to see where knowledge and skills are incorporated into specific courses. When educators know what knowledge and skills are being taught and where they are placed in the curriculum, educators can design courses that build on previous knowledge and skills.

EXAMPLES OF CURRICULUM MAPPING

Preliminary work on curriculum mapping has been accomplished through the identification of major nursing program concepts (organizing framework) and the leveling of educational outcomes by nursing program level, semester level, or patient education, or staff development learning program. It's now time to create a more-detailed curriculum map for the program or individual offering.

Table 8.1 builds on previous chapters and is one example of how to map the broader program curriculum. Since the level outcomes were used to guide the curricular map, congruency with the mission/philosophy statements, organizing framework, and educational outcomes of the program and practice standards for the discipline should have been maintained. Congruency has been demonstrated and presented in previous tables; therefore, it is not necessary to keep repeating this information. Essential knowledge and competencies need to be identified for all level outcomes.

Nursing Program Curriculum Mapping Worksheet

The example in Table 8.1 will assist educators in mapping the curriculum for a nursing program or an individual offering while maintaining congruency with the program mission/philosophy and organizing framework and with the organization/parent institution's mission and philosophy.

The simplest way to approach the task of mapping the curriculum is to use the major organizing concepts and the level outcomes developed in previous chapters.

1. Create a table with sufficient columns for all level outcomes.
2. Distribute the **Nursing Program Curriculum Mapping Worksheet** to all educators, requesting each educator list all subconcepts and content for each level that contributes to the learners' achievement of the stated level outcome. Remember the focus is not on content but

on what learners must know, understand, and/or do to achieve the outcome.

3. Collect and compile all educator subconcepts and content lists and share the master worksheet with all participants.

4. The educators should discuss all proposed subconcepts and content on the master worksheet and agree on consistency with the major concept, whether the difficulty level is appropriate for the level/learner outcome or if the level/learner outcome needs to be revised.

5. If additional concepts are identified at this time that are not in the program's organizing framework, it may be necessary to return to all previous program documents for revision.

6. Finalize the list of subconcepts and content, creating a comprehensive list that identifies the necessary knowledge and competencies learners must accomplish in order to meet the stated level/learner outcomes.

7. Place the comprehensive list in a new table and distribute to all educators. The comprehensive list will guide educators in developing courses that assist learners in meeting the stated level/learner outcome.

8. If courses already exist, comparing the comprehensive list to what is currently being taught should identify gaps, redundancies, and level of difficulty issues.

9. At this point, some educators may prefer developing concept maps that show the relationships between concepts and subconcepts and how they link the curriculum together within a course, semester, professional year, and/or the entire program.

10. By reading the table from left to right, you can quickly determine if a concept is being addressed adequately to achieve the stated level outcome and develops the necessary foundation for the learner to meet subsequent level outcomes.

TABLE 8.1 Example of Program Mapping With Two Levels

Organizing Concept With Corresponding Educational Outcome	Level 1	Level 2
Educational Outcome: Communication End-of-program performance and knowledge expectation.	Beginning performance/knowledge necessary to progress to Level 2. **Knowledge:** List necessary knowledge areas required for success. Subconcepts identified earlier should be incorporated here. **Competencies:** List necessary skills required for success.	Additional performance/knowledge necessary to meet Level 2 outcomes, thus meeting educational outcomes. **Knowledge:** List necessary knowledge areas required for success. **Competencies:** List necessary skills required for success.
Educational Outcome: Critical Thinking End-of-program performance and knowledge expectation.	Beginning performance/knowledge necessary to progress to Level 2. **Knowledge:** List necessary knowledge areas required for success. Subconcepts identified earlier should be incorporated here. **Competencies:** List necessary skills required for success.	Additional performance/knowledge necessary to meet Level 2 outcomes, thus meeting educational outcomes. **Knowledge:** List necessary knowledge areas required for success. **Competencies:** List necessary skills required for success.

Educational Outcome:
Mathematical Computation
End-of-program performance and knowledge expectation.

Beginning performance/knowledge necessary to progress to Level 2.

Knowledge:
List necessary knowledge areas required for success. Subconcepts identified earlier should be incorporated here.

Competencies:
List necessary skills required for success.

Additional performance/knowledge necessary to meet Level 2 outcomes, thus meeting educational outcomes.

Knowledge:
List necessary knowledge areas required for success.

Competencies:
List necessary skills required for success.

Educational Outcome: Person
End-of-program performance and knowledge expectation.

Beginning performance/knowledge necessary to progress to Level 2.

Knowledge:
List necessary knowledge areas required for success. Subconcepts identified earlier should be incorporated here.

Competencies:
List necessary skills required for success.

Additional performance/knowledge necessary to meet Level 2 outcomes, thus meeting educational outcomes.

Knowledge:
List necessary knowledge areas required for success.

Competencies:
List necessary skills required for success.

(continued)

TABLE 8.1 Example of Program Mapping With Two Levels *(continued)*

Organizing Concept With Corresponding Educational Outcome	Level 1	Level 2
Educational Outcome: Environment End-of-program performance and knowledge expectation.	Beginning performance/knowledge necessary to progress to Level 2. **Knowledge:** List necessary knowledge areas required for success. Subconcepts identified earlier should be incorporated here. **Competencies:** List necessary skills required for success.	Additional performance/knowledge necessary to meet Level 2 outcomes, thus meeting educational outcomes. **Knowledge:** List necessary knowledge areas required for success. **Competencies:** List necessary skills required for success.
Educational Outcome: Nursing End-of-program performance and knowledge expectation.	Beginning performance/knowledge necessary to progress to Level 2. **Knowledge:** List necessary knowledge areas required for success. Subconcepts identified earlier should be incorporated here. **Competencies:** List necessary skills required for success.	Additional performance/knowledge necessary to meet Level 2 outcomes, thus meeting educational outcomes. **Knowledge:** List necessary knowledge areas required for success. **Competencies:** List necessary skills required for success.

Educational Outcome: Health

End-of-program performance and knowledge expectation.

Beginning performance/knowledge necessary to progress to Level 2.

Knowledge:
List necessary knowledge areas required for success. Subconcepts identified earlier should be incorporated here.

Competencies:
List necessary skills required for success.

Additional performance/knowledge necessary to meet Level 2 outcomes, thus meeting educational outcomes.

Knowledge:
List necessary knowledge areas required for success.

Competencies:
List necessary skills required for success.

Educational Outcome: Teaching/learning

End-of-program performance and knowledge expectation.

Beginning performance/knowledge necessary to progress to Level 2.

Knowledge:
List necessary knowledge areas required for success. Subconcepts identified earlier should be incorporated here.

Competencies:
List necessary skills required for success.

Additional performance/knowledge necessary to meet Level 2 outcomes, thus meeting educational outcomes.

Knowledge:
List necessary knowledge areas required for success.

Competencies:
List necessary skills required for success.

Consistent with systems thinking, curricular maps are dependent on previous program elements and may need to be adjusted depending on changes in internal factors (e.g., changes in mission/philosophy statements with either the organization or program, changes in the organizing framework or the educational outcomes) and external factors (e.g., changes in practice standards, approval/accrediting standards, employer expectations); therefore, the curricular maps require periodic review. Once the "big picture" of mapping the curriculum has been completed, program courses need to be developed or existing courses revised so they are consistent with the broader curricular map. Learner outcomes for each course must contribute to the accomplishment of the level outcomes. As new or revised courses are added to the curricular map, the focus becomes narrower with the identification of detailed knowledge and competencies required for learners to accomplish the course outcomes.

Faculty are typically responsible for program/curriculum activities; therefore, faculty development is an important element for creating and managing successful nursing programs. The next chapter will explore the importance of faculty development activities to ensure program success.

9

Faculty Development
for Program Change

INTRODUCTION

An essential element in nursing program development or revision is to assist faculty to gain the knowledge and skills they need to carry out their responsibilities. All faculty and staff, as well as administrators, will have a part in program development. Faculty development is continuous because of all the changes, new processes, and ways of looking at nursing program content and processes. Successful program development or revision is dependent on faculty who are committed, willing to expand their perspective, appreciate acknowledgment for their efforts, and know they have gained new skills.

Faculty development continues with each new activity to further develop programs and make revisions as needed.

In this chapter, you will learn:

1. The purposes of faculty development related to curriculum development and revision.
2. How to prepare for resistance to change and new approaches.
3. Strategies to facilitate faculty development.

PURPOSES OF FACULTY DEVELOPMENT

Faculty development generally focuses on two areas: personal and professional growth related to their own goals and work-related expectations. Faculty members have areas of expertise such as clinical specializations and certification. Nurses come to educational settings with prior experience and have to become proficient in teaching, faculty responsibilities, and student interactions.

A starting place, to gain knowledge and skill in curriculum development, is to build on a nurse's existing critical thinking, analytic, organizational, technical, and practical skills. Faculty development, related to curriculum development, is extensive and includes all the essential institutional and nursing program elements.

To achieve the goals of faculty development for curriculum change, there has to be an awareness of changing roles and teaching approaches. Faculty need to actively participate in their own development, seek specific opportunities, and be prepared for change (Iwasiw, Goldenberg, & Andrusyszyn, 2009).

FAST FACTS in a NUTSHELL

- The main focus of faculty development is professional development for program development and revision.
- Faculty development activities build on nurses' previous specialized knowledge and skills.
- Skills for program development and revision include critical thinking and organizational ability.
- Faculty, individually, have to be aware of their development needs and seek opportunities.

ESSENTIAL ELEMENTS TO PREPARE FACULTY FOR CHANGE

Nursing faculty are responsible for program development and revision to meet accreditation standards and to keep content current. Program elements are usually updated when there are changes in institutional documents, external accrediting requirements, and revisions to textbooks. Faculty may not look for opportunities to change a program until there are specific requirements.

New faculty members are not prepared to take leadership responsibilities for program change. They may have new ideas and approaches but often meet resistance from experienced faculty. Nursing program leaders keep current with required standards, requirements for new specializations, and changes in health care that impact nursing education.

The challenge to successfully implement change is to understand faculty behaviors related to change. Lewin's theory addresses the need for nursing program leaders and faculty to identify why change is needed (unfreezing phase). The forces that are driving or may restrain the change (force field analysis) are explored (moving phase). The actions required to make the changes are carried out. Finally, the changes are stabilized (refreezing phase) in both the individuals and the system (Iwasiw et al., 2009).

The Transtheoretical Model of Behavior Change focuses on different stages of change for individuals. The ability and willingness of individuals to change attitudes, intentions, and behaviors are critical to faculty development. It is important to understand that some faculty will not see the need for change (precontemplation stage). Faculty may think (contemplation phase) about the positive and negative aspects of change but are not ready to act. When faculty begin to plan making changes (preparation phase), they are ready to participate in faculty development activities and to make small changes.

In the action phase, faculty are committed to change and are ready to learn the new skills required. Once the changes are made, faculty need to continue (maintenance phase) with the new approaches and avoid going back to previous attitudes, intentions, and behaviors (Iwasiw et al., 2009). Table 9.1 summarizes change theories.

From our nursing experiences, we know that many colleagues and patients do not change their behaviors. Rogers (1983) researched how new ideas are shared and adopted in all types of settings (Diffusion of Innovation Theory). He found the primary factors that support the adoption of changes are the characteristics of the adopters, the innovation, and the change agents.

In nursing education, the students are often the adopters of new processes and technologies. Faculty are diverse and may adopt change quickly, adopt some change, or not want any change. Everyone has adopted the innovations of using

TABLE 9.1 Examples of Change Theories/Models

Lewin's force field analysis	Change is a social-psychological process and has three phases: unfreezing, moving, and refreezing (Iwasiw et al., 2009).
Diffusion of innovation theory	Examines the processes about how innovations are adopted by individuals and organizations (Rogers, 1983).
Transtheoretical Model of Behavior Change	Individual behavior changes include alterations in attitudes, intentions, and behaviors. The change process steps allow individuals to go back and forth between each step and finally maintain new behaviors (Iwasiw et al., 2009).

computers and the Internet, on different levels. The more abstract or the more difficult an innovation is, the fewer people will adopt it early. In nursing education, there is continuing discussion about the use of simulation for clinical experiences. Change agents, such as deans or nursing directors, have the formal power to initiate change. Informal leaders, who have knowledge and experience, can be role models for their peers. The culture of a nursing education or clinical practice setting is regularly exposed to change, but members also want to continue with what they are currently doing.

Rogers (1983) found that about 2% to 3% of people (innovators) in an organization are quick to adopt new ideas and practices. They may not be trusted by others because they move so quickly and are not concerned about stabilizing changes. The next group (early adopters) represent about 10% to 15% of a group and feel positive about change. The early majority (30% to 35%) of a group can be persuaded by others to adopt change. The late majority adopters (30% to 35%) of a group are unconvinced to adopt new ideas until they can clearly see the benefits. The last group comprises the laggards (10% to 20%), who are not open to changes and may actively resist the introduction of new ideas (Rogers, 1983).

In any nursing education setting, there are differences in how faculty and staff are ready to make changes. It is important to understand these differences in order to determine specific faculty development opportunities and to know that some faculty may not respond to changes for a long time, or ever.

Many of the changes in nursing education are related to the use and application of technology and collection of data for program improvement. This can be very challenging for nurse educators and for the leaders to plan faculty development programs.

======================================*FAST FACTS in a NUTSHELL*

- Faculty have the major responsibility of developing and revising nursing education programs.
- Use theories/models as a framework to plan for faculty development.
- Gaining an understanding of why change is needed is a first step.
- Understanding faculty attitudes, intentions, and behaviors is essential to planning faculty development activities.
- Become aware of individual faculty responses to change.

In any nursing education setting, despite efforts to create change, faculty and staff may resist. There are two common forms of resistance.

Active (overt) resistance to change is demonstrated in different ways:

- Direct criticism of the proposed changes and faculty development plans
- Not accepting the need for change
- Predicting dire consequences of program development and revision activities
- Directly refusing to participate in faculty development events

Passive (covert) resistance is displayed when individuals do not openly state opposition:

- Miss or arrive late for meetings
- Limited participation in meetings
- Not completing assigned tasks
- Creating diversions when interacting with others by changing or bringing up different topics

Nurse leaders have the responsibility to address resistance directly through:

- Private meetings with individuals
- Listening to resisters so they know they are heard
- Stating expectations clearly about their responsibilities to participate
- Publicly demonstrating behaviors that reflect the goals for faculty development
- Sharing consequences of not participating in faculty development and supporting program goals (Iwasiw et al., 2009).

Nurse leaders need to carefully determine the best fit for each faculty, based on their specific characteristics. Creating faculty teams, with different approaches to change, promote learning and sharing of expertise. All faculty need to participate at some level. Faculty development resources should be directed to the faculty and areas that will make the biggest differences in meeting the goals of program development and revision.

FAST FACTS in a NUTSHELL

- Resistance to change is a frequent human response.
- Active resistance to change is demonstrated by overt verbal and nonverbal negative responses and behaviors.
- Passive resistance to change is demonstrated by covert behaviors resulting in not accomplishing tasks.
- Nurse leaders need to address both active and passive resistance to change.
- Nurse leaders have the responsibility to find best fits for each faculty member to ensure everyone is participating.

Definition of Key Terms
- **Force field analysis** is a technique for looking at all the forces for and against a plan. It helps to evaluate the importance of these factors and decide if a plan is worth implementing (from www.mindtools.com/pages/article/newTED_06.htm).

KEY POINTS

Faculty have the major responsibility to develop, monitor, and improve nursing education programs. To carry out this responsibility, they need to learn new information and accept that change is needed. Nurse leaders, in all educational settings, need to recognize resistance to change, address it, and help faculty move forward in the change processes. Strategies to facilitate changes, that meet the goals of the program changes, are needed to achieve success.

========*FAST FACTS in a NUTSHELL*

- Change is an ongoing process in nursing education programs.
- All faculty need to participate at some level.
- The nursing leaders, in the educational setting, set the culture and tone for change.
- Specific faculty development plans support success.

EXAMPLES OF FACULTY DEVELOPMENT PLANS

Faculty development plans are formed in many different ways to meet the needs of an educational setting or organization. The following examples are from published articles and illustrate different types of faculty development projects.

Loving, G. L., & Wilson, J. S. (2000). Infusing critical thinking into the nursing curriculum through faculty development. *Nurse Educator,* 25(2), 70–75.

Abstract: An important prerequisite to changes in an educational program's predominant philosophy and culture is systematic faculty development to begin and sustain the evolution. The authors describe how one nursing school implemented a faculty development program with the goal of infusing critical thinking strategies into courses throughout the curriculum.

Latimer, D. G., & Thornlow, D. K. (2006). Incorporating geriatrics into baccalaureate nursing curricula: Laying the groundwork with faculty development. *Journal of Professional Nursing,* 22(3), 79–83.

Abstract: In June 2001, the John A. Hartford Foundation of New York awarded the American Association of Colleges of Nursing (AACN) a $3.99 million grant to enhance gerontology curriculum development and new clinical experiences in 20 baccalaureate and 10 graduate schools of nursing. Faculty development is the single most necessary precursor to the successful implementation and maintenance of geriatric curricular enhancements. Unless faculty members foster positive attitudes toward aging, expand their geriatric nursing knowledge base, and are able to integrate geriatric content into the curricula, progress cannot be made.

Jarrett, S., Horner, M., Center, D., & Kane, L. A. (2008). Curriculum for the development of staff nurses as clinical faculty and scholars. *Nurse Educator,* 33(6), 268–272.

Abstract: The authors describe a unique educational program developed collaboratively in numerous educational and practice institutions to prepare staff nurses to assume a teaching role. A wide variety of teaching strategies were presented and demonstrated in the course so that the participants acquired new knowledge and skills to implement the clinical faculty role. This new pool of clinical faculty completed the course with a defined skill set and the title of clinical scholar.

Curran, C. R. (2008). Faculty development initiatives for the integration of informatics competencies and point-of-care technologies in undergraduate nursing education. *Nursing Clinics of North America, 43*(4), 523–533.

Abstract: Faculty members have a critical role in deciding the content that is taught to their nursing students. They must grasp the importance of using technology to facilitate learning and knowledge of informatics concepts and skills. This article describes a successful faculty development program that was aimed at upgrading the technology and informatics skills of the faculty while at the same time developing and threading informatics skills across the baccalaureate nursing curriculum.

FAST FACTS in a NUTSHELL

Faculty development programs are diverse and organized to meet the needs of faculty to manage change. Development activities and projects may focus on:

- Adding new concepts into a nursing program.
- Arranging activities for faculty to teach new content to students.
- Educating clinical nurses for new roles.
- Preparing faculty so they are ready to teach new skills to students.

Changes in health and nursing care make it essential to develop nurses so they have current knowledge, skills, and attitudes to meet practice and professional standards and expectations.

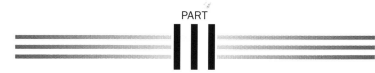

PART

III

Curriculum and Course Design

10

Elements of a Curriculum

INTRODUCTION

A curriculum is a comprehensive collection of statements that usually include a mission, vision, and philosophy. Faculty beliefs about teaching, learning, nursing, health, person, diversity, and environment are included. A conceptual framework organizes the curriculum information. Details related to these topics were covered in earlier chapters.

Undergraduate nursing programs are offered at different levels and have similarities but also differences. Graduate nursing programs are also offered at different levels. New nursing curricula are developed when degrees and/or specializations are planned. Revisions to existing nursing curricula are made as standards, guidelines, regulations, and health care environments change.

In this chapter, you will learn:

1. Purposes of a curriculum.
2. Elements of a curriculum.
3. Selected factors that influence curriculum development processes.

PURPOSES OF A CURRICULUM

Nursing programs of study need to be dynamic and be ready to adapt to changes in regulations, standards, education, and nursing practice. Nursing curricula have different purposes. All stakeholders; educators, practicing nurses, and health care institutions need to organize and implement the concepts and content that prepare learners to function in the diverse and changing health care environment. Another purpose is to respond to changing population and environmental patterns. Nurse educators should also incorporate input from consumers, students, and nursing leaders to maintain relevance (Keating, 2010). A final purpose is to identify how a curriculum addresses quality, accessibility, and economic soundness (Billings & Halstead, 2008).

================*FAST FACTS in a NUTSHELL*

- Nursing curricula are dynamic to stay current.
- Addressing health care and population shifts is essential.
- Input from wide audiences supports creating/revising a curriculum that is inclusive.
- Information about quality and cost of nursing programs is part of the purposes.

ELEMENTS OF A CURRICULUM

Chapters 1 through 5 covered the foundational documents required for developing a nursing curriculum. Once it is determined how the nursing program foundational documents fit with the institution/organization mission, philosophy, and educational outcomes, the specific curriculum elements are determined or revised.

A nursing program mission is linked to the institution/ organization and includes specific elements such as:

- Educating graduates to meet the health needs of a diverse population
- Preparing nurses who are caring and competent
- Participating in service learning to improve the health and welfare of communities
- Preparing graduates for advanced education and continued professional development

An organizing framework is based on selected models or theories. Typically, three learning domains are included: cognitive, affective, and psychomotor. Common nursing program frameworks are:

- Orem's Theory of Self Care
- Peplau's Theory of Interpersonal Relationships
- Leininger's Theory of Cultural Care
- Watson's Human Science and Caring

Learning theories may be used to organize a curriculum and to identify values and beliefs about learning processes. Examples of learning theories are:

- Behaviorism is based on the idea that teaching is achieved by learners achieving the observable, measurable, and controllable objectives determined by teachers.
- Cognitivism addresses the need to individualize learning so all students are successful.
- Humanism focuses on the development of self that will advance thinking and learning.
- Constructivism theory identifies that learners have prior knowledge and experience to support new learning.

- Organizational learning is based on the theory that all humans want to learn and organizations need to encourage the social aspects of learning: teams and interdependent projects (Keating, 2010).

FAST FACTS in a NUTSHELL

- A nursing program mission sets the direction for content, activities, and outcomes.
- Nursing and related theories and models provide specific directions for nursing curricula.
- Learning theories serve as a basis for selecting teaching/ learning strategies.

CURRICULUM GOALS

Curriculum goals are statements about the expected attributes and competencies of graduates. Statements include philosophical guiding principles, curriculum guidelines, and the expected outcomes. Goals may also be referred to as terminal objectives.

Curriculum goals are part of the published program documents and include all audiences: faculty, students, employers, and other members of the institution/organization and external groups (accrediting bodies, professional groups, and the public) (Iwasiw, Goldenberg, & Andrusyszyn, 2009).

DIFFERENT TYPES OF CURRICULA

The official curriculum elements are derived from the program documents (mission, philosophy, framework, etc.). The operational curriculum is what is taught by the faculty who stress the importance of selected content. The hidden curriculum is communicated through faculty verbal and nonverbal behaviors. Students pick up on these behaviors related to interactions, teaching strategies, and class priorities. The null curriculum consists of what is not taught. Faculty need to be aware of what they are not teaching and why (Billings & Halsted, 2008).

Curriculum development is a planned process that needs effort and commitment from the faculty, nursing administration, and institution. Visionary leadership sets the culture for curriculum development. Curriculum development is part of planned change in a nursing program. Including development processes in faculty meetings and committees promotes efficiency and effectiveness. Because of rapid changes in standards, regulations, and the health care environments, curriculum development must move forward as quickly as possible to be current (Billings & Halsted, 2008).

═══════════════════════════════*FAST FACTS in a NUTSHELL*

- Faculty and teachers need to be aware of the different types of curricula so they can blend the best of each type into the curriculum changes.
- Excellent planning and organization of the curriculum development processes help the goals in a timely manner.
- Be aware of all the regulations, standards, guidelines, and future health care system changes so the development work includes these elements.

CURRICULUM DEVELOPMENT PROCESSES

Determine who can provide the leadership to influence people and will have hands-on involvement, be competent, and trustworthy. Effective leaders possess the knowledge, skills, and attitudes essential for curriculum development. Select a committee/

working group structure so there is broad involvement initially and then smaller working groups to complete tasks.

A detailed work plan facilitates achieving the goals in the expected timeframe. Develop an in-house project plan or use commercial software project planning tools. Secure the financial, environmental, and human resources needed to complete the project.

Accurate and detailed record keeping and sharing of information are essential. Everyone involved wants to keep updated about what is happening, provide their input at strategic times, and know their roles and responsibilities (Iwasiw et al., 2009).

FAST FACTS in a NUTSHELL

- Nursing education new program development or revision of an existing program is complex and needs broad-based financial and human resources to achieve the stated goals.
- Having a very detailed project plan helps to identify and track each step.

FACTORS INFLUENCING CURRICULUM DEVELOPMENT

External influences that affect nursing program curriculum development relate to global social and health issues, national political health-related issues, shifting demographics, explosion of technology, and environmental changes.

Nursing curricula need to address the global issues that impact nursing practice. These could include lack of basic human needs such as clean water and diseases that result from poverty and social upheavals.

We are all aware of the major changes approved or proposed in the United States. Nursing curricula need to include strategies to keep current as issues evolve.

There are demographic shifts throughout the world and within countries. In the United States, major demographic changes include an increasingly older population, diversity of cultural groups, and immigration. Nursing curricula need strategies to include new content within a current framework.

Some environmental changes may impact populations for decades and others are sudden events that totally disrupt individuals and groups.

Internal factors include institutional financial and human resource allocation, availability of clinical sites, and the need for additional faculty and staff to support a new program or additional specialization in an existing program.

FAST FACTS in a NUTSHELL

- Curriculum development processes in nursing education must take into account the external factors that impact the type of program.
- The project plan should include how and where the external factors will be addressed.
- Internal factors have a major impact on the actual approval and development/revision of a nursing education program.
- Finding answers and support at the beginning of the project is essential.

Definition of Key Terms
- A **curriculum** is a comprehensive collection of statements related to major program elements.
- **Curriculum** goals are broad statements that identify the curriculum elements and expected learner outcomes for all interested groups.
- A **program model** describes how a curriculum is organized.

KEY POINTS

Nursing program curricula in the United States have common purposes because of the many levels and types of internal and external regulations, standards, and guidelines. Nursing educators have shared values and beliefs about education. Purposes are refined to be congruent with the values and beliefs of the organization in which they reside.

Nursing program curricula have very similar elements, derived from the internal and external regulations, standards, and guidelines. Specific elements are related to the degree levels, particular certification, and audiences.

There are many internal and external factors that impact the development of each curriculum. They include the ones identified earlier in this chapter but also need to refer to changes in health care environments both nationally and globally.

EXAMPLES OF CURRICULUM DEVELOPMENT

There are many different approaches to curriculum development. The nursing faculty at Central College were asked to develop a new specialization in the master's program with a focus on informatics.

Use Current Resources and Processes

The curriculum committee structure worked well, except they had not planned any new programs. The current curriculum tasks were being done. Tasks were reassigned with expanded faculty and staff participation to meet the new challenges. Faculty with leadership potential were selected to head subcommittees.

Consultation

The faculty, teaching in the MSN program, needed additional expertise to develop the program. During the initial program planning meeting, a budget was developed. It included funds for a consultant who currently directed an informatics specialization.

Educational Resources

Current faculty also wanted to learn more about curriculum development processes. They found different websites with resources.

The National League for Nursing (NLN) has several resources for curriculum development. Faculty programs and resources include:

- The annual NLN Education Summit, a conference and show attracting 2000 nurse educators
- Conferences on specific topics like technology, nursing education research, and leadership development
- The annual Immersion Experience, where faculty spend a week engaged with experts in a specific area of nursing education
- Regional workshops, often co-sponsored with state constituent leagues, member schools, or other nursing organizations
- Webinars, the lowest-cost series that brings programs to the school via the Web and a speaker phone (www.nln .org/facultyprograms/index.htm)

Organizational Resources

The chairperson of the nursing curriculum committee met with the college curriculum chair person to review the steps in the process and to determine what resources were available. The college uses a project planning software package to input and track all the steps. The staff also provided training and support.

Evidence-Based Research

The faculty team responsible for developing the program worked with the college librarian to search for research-based information to use when developing the new informatics specialization. The following is an example of a research article.

A problem-based learning model for nursing curriculum development challenges teachers to become facilitators and learners to become self-directed. Content is selected from nursing practice. The limitations and strengths of different curriculum development models are presented and compared to a problem-based model (from Practice to Theory: Reconceptualising Curriculum Development for Problem Based Learning. www.tp.edu.sg/pbl_janeconway-pennylittle.pdf).

Regulatory, Approval Standards/ Guidelines

The faculty team responsible for pulling together the last nursing program accreditation visit met and reviewed current standards for National League for Nursing accreditation standards (2011). They developed a summary of all the information required for each standard and shared it with everyone involved in developing the new specialization.

FAST FACTS in a NUTSHELL

- Maximize current structures, processes, and resources for program development.
- Select a consultant who has the skill and knowledge to get the project started.
- Select educational resources to help faculty and staff gain knowledge about curriculum development.
- Use organizational resources to fit project into the common expectations.
- Review evidence and best practices related to curriculum development and the specialization.
- Use current information to assure the new specialization meets approval regulations, guidelines, and standards.

11

Elements of Curriculum Design

INTRODUCTION

There are many parts to designing nursing education curricula. The previous chapters provided the foundation information to build and design a curriculum. The limits of the design, moving processes forward, delivery options, and sequencing of courses are all considered. Curriculum design is presented as a sequential process but it is also creative. Ideas are exchanged, debated, and agreed upon. Faculty and other stakeholders also have input (Iwasiw, Goldenberg, & Andrusyszyn, 2009).

In this chapter, you will learn:

1. The common elements and processes for designing a curriculum.
2. To recognize different types of curriculum designs.
3. To select delivery approaches.
4. To determine appropriate organizing structures to support curriculum design.

PURPOSES OF A NURSING PROGRAM CURRICULUM

The purposes of a nursing program curriculum include using the agreed-on mission, philosophy, and organizing framework to develop the overall goals of the program. Nursing faculty need to create a plan to place content throughout the curriculum. Another purpose is to address health care needs of society and of persons with specific disease conditions. Finally, determine the competencies and outcomes for graduates of the program.

Definition of Key Terms
- **Curriculum design processes** are all the activities related to creating or revising curricula.
- **Curriculum types** are related to the program goals and determine the number of courses and learning activities.
- **Curriculum structure** refers to how programs are arranged.
- **Program delivery** is how the curriculum is presented to the learners.
- **Stakeholders** are the internal and external individuals, groups, and organizations that have an interest in ensuring graduates are prepared for nursing practice.

KEY POINTS

Because there are so many parts to designing a curriculum, the boundaries or limits must be discussed and determined. The design is often affected by the realities of both internal and external contextual elements. Program designers will have information such as the availability of faculty, institutional/organizational policies and resources, support for non-traditional teaching/learning approaches, and partnerships. External contextual elements include accreditation, professional approval, and regulatory standards and guidelines.

The curriculum design process needs to be comprehensive and include all the processes required. Seek input from colleagues in similar programs. It can be an option to hire a consultant to provide expertise. Review documents that include institutional/organizational policies and board of nursing, accreditation, and professional requirements. It is very helpful to use all these resources during the design process (Iwasi et al., 2009). For example, certain content and the number of clinical hours may be specified by an approval agency.

A draft plan could include semester and course listings, credit allocation, sequencing of content, and lab and clinical experiences. This is an important step in which to include stakeholders so they can point out difficulties and offer improvements. For example, the length of the program is tied to financial aid and cost. Is it possible to complete the program in the expected time? What additions and changes are needed to provide nonnursing courses? What clinical resources are currently available, and how is it possible to expand or contract the number and type of them? These elements are all part of designing a curriculum.

═══════════════════════*FAST FACTS in a NUTSHELL*

- Designing a curriculum is a complex process.
- Creating a plan facilitates the design process.
- Seek outside sources and information to start the processes.
- Consider all the different elements needed to design a curriculum so it is complete and useful for everyone involved.

Curriculum designs are tied to the type and level of nursing programs. Faculty need to design programs that support the selected goals, outcomes, and competencies that are congruent with the foundational documents.

Curricular designs also address mobility and "ladders" between the different levels of nursing education. In community colleges, there are curricula that prepare licensed vocational nurses to move to associate degree nursing programs. Associate degree graduates can also move to baccalaureate and master's programs with articulation agreements at colleges and universities. Nursing curricula designs can also address the needs of students with non-nursing degrees and international students to enter and be successful in nursing programs by taking into account their previous knowledge and experiences.

FAST FACTS in a NUTSHELL

- A curriculum design must show how it flows from the mission, philosophy, and program outcomes.
- There is great diversity in nursing programs, and curriculum designs need to be congruent with the different types and levels.
- Learners' previous knowledge and experience must be considered in the design processes.
- Internal/external constraints affect a curriculum design.

Traditional curricula may be designed with content blocked, sequenced, threaded, or integrated. This approach has been and is still used when program delivery is in structured settings with face-to-face classes scheduled. By the end of a program, students will meet the requirements from each course and therefore the program expectations. Contemporary designs use a variety of design approaches that still offer traditional elements but also use other ways to present content.

Within contemporary designs there are still options to organize content in a traditional way.

One curriculum design is a competency-based approach. Competency-based education (CBE) begins with the end in mind. The main focus is always on the outcome or end results, rather than the processes. All the assessments in a program are tied to the identified competencies. Learners have the opportunity to study and learn until they demonstrate competency in specific areas. Carrie Lenberg developed an approach to CBE with her Competency Outcomes and Performance Assessment (COPA) Model (Anema & McCoy, 2010).

A problem-based learning curriculum design supports active student participation related to identifying problems. A case study approach challenges learners to discuss problems and use prior knowledge and skills to resolve them (Lowenstein & Bradshaw, 2007). In addition to written case studies, there are commercial projects available that focus on simulations and games to encourage active learning and problem solving.

Nursing programs, for many years, were delivered by face-to-face instruction in classrooms, skills laboratories, and clinical settings. Other types of education, for staff nurses, patients, and consumers, were carried out in the same way. Advantages to the traditional delivery of education are that faculty can physically be with learners, interact with them, communicate with each other, and resolve any issues.

Programs, in the past, delivered curricula by correspondence courses. This was a popular delivery approach for many years but is not common now. Learners receive materials by mail, complete assignments, and return them. They can be in contact with faculty via phone, fax, or the Internet. Distance education provides more advanced delivery approaches than correspondence courses.

We are all aware of distance education. Higher education, staff development, and patient education institutions/organizations have adopted this delivery approach in many settings and for all types of students. Traditional and totally online institutions/organizations usually have commercial, full service learning platforms that support all the teaching/learning activities needed for programs, except clinical experiences. Simulations are allowed to replace some on-site clinical experiences.

Other technology-based delivery approaches are well suited to meetings, collaboration with partners, and global contacts. Broadcast television is delivered through satellite and TV methods. Programs are viewed by learners in many different settings at the same time. Video and teleconferencing options allow participants to interact with each other, see each other, and view information. Computer conferencing is done in a shared space where faculty and learners communicate by typing messages to each other and responding. Attachments can also be shared (Iwasiw et al., 2009).

Partnerships with other institutions or commercial companies provide new opportunities for curricula to be offered in more than one location. For example, one graduate nursing program could be offered throughout a state or regional consortium arrangement. Commercial companies have developed many curriculum products to support teaching/learning. There are e-books and study guides, links to additional resources, practice assessments, and discussions. Hybrid approaches are considered based on resources, availability of educational materials, and the diversity of learners (age, location, culture, language, and educational needs) (Iwasiw et al., 2009). With so many curriculum design options, faculty need to select a range of approaches that are congruent with the institution/organization and meets learner needs.

Florence Nightingale's curriculum structure focused on environment. Structures have evolved since that time to provide organization and order in nursing programs.

==*FAST FACTS in a NUTSHELL*

- Nursing curriculum structures have evolved since Florence Nightingale started modern nursing with a focus on environment.
- Explore the features of both traditional and contemporary curriculum structures.
- Technology has made a huge impact on how nursing curricula are structured.
- Consider hybrid structures to accommodate all the different elements needed to achieve program outcomes.

Nursing education program structures have evolved and continue to change. Traditional organizing approaches include:

- A *medical model* is organized around diseases related to body systems. This model fits with nursing education programs in hospital settings.
- A *simple to complex* structure organizes knowledge and content sequentially. The curriculum may start with individuals, move to families, and then communities.
- *Stages of illness* may start with maintaining health, acute care, rehabilitation, and chronic care.

Contemporary organizing approaches focus on:

- Conceptual frameworks, models, and theories to define nursing concepts in the program content and learning activities.

- Organizing a curriculum according to outcomes is promoted by accrediting bodies.
- Typical outcomes center on cognitive skills, personal and professional development, interdisciplinary team skills, and the knowledge, attitudes, and skills essential for safe and quality nursing practice (Iwasiw et al., 2009).

With the acceleration of change in health care, nursing education curriculum will also change. Health care providers will have a greater voice in determining how to prepare graduates to be ready for practice. The need to practice within interdisciplinary teams will require collaborative courses with other disciplines. Options for career mobility and articulation between nursing programs will impact curriculum designs.

Nursing education programs will also develop and offer programs for staff development, patient education, and consumer information (Billings & Halsted, 2008). Curriculum design is a dynamic process and faculty need to be ready to share responsibility, gather information from many sources, and make design choices as indicated.

EXAMPLES OF NURSING PROGRAM CURRICULUM DESIGNS

A Career Ladder/Curriculum Design at Muskegon Community College. (2011). Retrieved October 30, 2011, from www.muskegoncc.edu/pages/572.asp

A PPT presentation for Designing a New Nursing Curriculum: The Process. (2011). Retrieved October 30, 2011, from www.nc-net.info/2006conf/Nursing_curric.ppt

The master's program in nursing reflects the core values and the tradition of liberal arts education at Goshen College. The curriculum design is compatible with standards outlined by the National Organization of Nurse Practitioner Faculties.

Developing a competency-based curriculum in HIV for nursing schools in Haiti. (2011). Retrieved October 30, 2011, from www.human-resources-health.com/content/6/1/17 (Human Resources for Health 2008;6:17 full-text article)

A Nursing Education Certification curriculum track at Texas Woman's University

College of Nursing developed a post-master's education-focused track. This track is designed for students who hold a master's degree in nursing (MS or MSN) with a defined clinical specialty focus of study. The purpose of the track is to prepare educators to assume positions in the areas of staff development, continuing education, or academia (2011). Retrieved October 30, 2011, from www.twu.edu/nursing/nursing-education-certification.asp

12

Elements of Course Design

INTRODUCTION

Courses need to match the elements approved for the curriculum and also build on the program and institutional/organizational foundational documents. Course designs are selected based on existing courses or the opportunity to include new options to achieve the outcomes. The wide variety of course options may make it difficult to select the essential elements of a course. Because there is so much information, multiple requirements, and diverse types of programs, it is a challenge in nursing education to be selective and design courses that are realistic and balanced.

In this chapter, you will learn:

1. The common elements and processes for designing a course.
2. To determine the internal and external factors that have an impact on course design.
3. To select different types of teaching strategies for course design.

PURPOSES OF COURSE DESIGN ELEMENTS

Each course has a purpose in a curriculum. A purpose statement makes it clear why and how that course fits. This aspect is important for learners to understand why they are taking a course and how it fits into a curriculum. A purpose statement also becomes part of the published information so prospective learners can examine a course.

The number and type of course credits are identified. Required hours for class, clinical, and laboratory experiences are listed. An expanded version of the purpose, with additional information, is placed in a syllabus or other course information (Iwasiw, Goldenberg, & Andrusyszyn, 2009).

═══════════════════════════════════*FAST FACTS in a NUTSHELL*

- A course design provides information about its purpose and how it fits within a curriculum.
- Course design processes select information to share expectations with learners.
- Specific course elements are determined as part of the design process.

Definition of Key Terms
- A **course** is a collection of content, teaching/learning activities, resources, and evaluation methods.
- **Course design** is the process of selecting all the course components.
- A **syllabus** contains all the essential course information.
- **Learning styles** refer to the different approaches individuals learn. Examples are visual, auditory, active, passive, abstract, and concrete.
- **Rounding points** means adding value to raise/lower decimals to whole numbers.

- **Weighting assignments** means assigning specific values to each assignment.
- **Teaching strategies** are the range of activities used by faculty to guide learning.

KEY POINTS

Course design processes are similar to curriculum design processes because they involve several steps of discussion, revision, and approvals before being finalized. Curriculum mapping was presented in Chapter 8 and provides a guide for making course decisions.

Select a course title that is descriptive and follows a pattern for the entire curriculum. Nursing course titles often identify the level of a course and major content, such as, Medical-Surgical Nursing 1 and 2, Critical Care Nursing, Community-Based Care, Evidence-Based Nursing Practice, or Legal/Ethical Principles for Nursing Practice. The first ideas for a course title provide direction for continued course design and may change as the process proceeds.

Develop a course description that is brief, comprehensive, and understandable and creates interest about the course content. Choose words carefully so the description is clear.

Focus the description on what the course is about. Begin the description with an eye-catching sentence (new information, interesting details, or results). Include the major content areas. You may use sentence fragments, such as *topics include* or *course includes* (specify content areas). Use action verbs: *discover, develop, apply, evaluate,* and *critique.*

Eliminate words that are obvious or implied: *this course introduces, focuses on, emphasizes, is the study of.* Academic course descriptions must be the same in all published information—university catalog, course offering lists, course syllabi, and any other documents. Courses offered for persons in a community could include wording about the benefits of taking a course. Course descriptions are about 50 to 100 words.

As described earlier, there are different approaches to curriculum design and this is also true for course design. Select a traditional, contemporary, or hybrid approach.

FAST FACTS in a NUTSHELL

- Use available resources, such as from other program elements, to build courses.
- Course descriptions are concise and informative.
- Review common types of course designs to determine the best fit for your program.

Determine which of the curriculum goals and outcomes are tied to each course. Chapter 7 describes the purposes of leveling outcomes. Each course has specific outcomes related to content and placement in the curriculum. This information is applied to clinical and laboratory nursing courses to ensure nurses provide safe and quality care. During this step, you need to realize that the course is one part of the total curriculum rather than trying to accomplish many outcomes.

FAST FACTS in a NUTSHELL

- Clearly demonstrate how courses are linked to curriculum goals and outcomes.
- Course content and outcomes are placed to fit within the overall curriculum plan.
- Compare all the courses to each other and to the total curriculum to determine overlap and gaps.

Selecting content is a challenging process because there is so much available. Discussing and sorting out what competencies you expect students to demonstrate at the end of the course and their congruency with program outcomes will start the process.

One of the main issues is the volume of content. For example, a medical-surgical text may have over 2,000 pages. Is it even possible to cover all that content in three or four courses?

Decisions about content are critical to student learning and success. Consider the following factors to determine content:

- Morbidity and mortality reports provide information about many different conditions.
- U.S. demographic patterns related to age, ethnicity, poverty, and geographic distribution.
- The clinical environment to focus on common conditions the students will experience.
- The levels of care offered in clinical settings, from a community hospital to a comprehensive medical and research center.

Process approaches, such as problem- and competency-based models and the nursing process in programs, allow for additions of content without changing curriculum and course elements.

Courses have set guidelines:

- The number of class sessions each term or semester
- Grouping content in a logical order for teaching and learning
- Emphasizing selected goals related to course content (Iwasiw et al., 2009)

═══════════════════════════════*FAST FACTS in a NUTSHELL*

- Recognize the need to carefully select content and separate "essential" from "nice to know."
- Use evidence about conditions and population demographics to help select content.
- Create course guidelines that are consistent with approved courses within the institution.

Select teaching strategies that fit with the purpose of a course and consider the learners' characteristics. Lecture is the most common method, with teachers controlling the content and its presentation.

Develop learner activities and include additional resources: multimedia, Internet, objects, and outside experts. Think about learning strategies to actively engage learners.

Incorporate case studies, role playing, and learner presentations. Distance education synchronous and asynchronous online discussions engage learners. Teleconferencing and online meetings support active learning. Creating videos of student presentations, interactions with others, and demonstration of skills is possible. Include multiple options to support and enhance learning.

Plan how to evaluate learners' outcomes. Select multiple methods to address different learning styles. Determine the advantages and disadvantages of methods based on your learning environment. Be sure evaluation is matched to course goals and supports program outcomes.

Clearly describe the grading system: weighting of assignments, points needed for letter grades, rounding points, options for improving grades, criteria assigned to pass/fail grades, and policies for missed tests or late papers. The outcomes of evaluation and the grades earned are very important to students. This is a topic that is often discussed by faculty and students as issues arise.

FAST FACTS in a NUTSHELL

- Select multiple evaluation methods to measure different types of outcomes.
- Assess the unique needs of diverse learners and those at a distance.
- Essential evaluation elements are consistency, reliability, and valid methods.

In the current educational and health care environments, there are many factors that impact nursing education. Nursing programs are offered within institutions/organizations and need to meet all expectations. Budgetary constraints are a concern for everyone. This means new full-time faculty are not hired, more adjunct faculty are hired, current faculty workloads are heavy, support staff is limited, and skills equipment is not replaced. Nurses are resourceful and can focus on working smarter and finding new ways to achieve course outcomes.

Analyze the number and types of assignments in each course. For example, if there are several written projects, how many are needed to ensure students have those skills? Is it possible to use simulations and laboratory experiences as part of clinical? How often do examinations, course materials, and learning resources need revisions? Seek outside funding to meet specific needs.

External factors include regulations that focus on student attrition, graduation, and financial aid outcomes. Educational institutions must meet all the regulations and provide documentation. Regional accrediting bodies also have extensive requirements. Nursing education programs have to meet all the institutional requirements as well as nursing accreditation and state requirements. Acceptable NCLEX-RN® pass rates are set by state boards of nursing with specific requirements if not met.

Course designs can support students achieving positive results. Review current practices, look at problem areas, determine best practices, and make changes as appropriate. Faculty have different approaches to implementing courses, but there have to be common approaches. For example, the faculty may agree on a format for a three-hour class session. The format includes lecture for background information and a focus on the nursing process applied to patient care. There is time for students to actively participate. In one class the format is followed. In another class a faculty spends most of the time lecturing about medical conditions with little time on application to patient care and not allowing student participation. In this class the faculty feels there is so much to learn and "crams" in too much information. Faculty accountability for delivering courses as intended is an essential consideration when designing courses.

In Chapter 11, the structure of a nursing program is described. Once that is determined, teaching strategies are selected to present the content. Include different teaching strategies to capture and hold learner interest. Learners cannot sit for two to three hours, even with short breaks, and focus on faculty lectures. Common options include:

- *Lecture,* which is useful to start a class by providing background information for complex concepts. It is a very efficient approach to cover a great deal of content in a short time.
- *Debates* support learner participation with presentation of conflicting opinions about nursing and health care issues.
- *Case studies,* based on patient conditions and nursing practice decisions, require critical analysis and link theory to practice. The outcomes reflect the prior decisions and learners can revise their decisions to achieve different outcomes.
- *Collaborative learning* requires teams/groups to work on projects. This approach enhances interdisciplinary learning opportunities and promotes listening, communication, and organizational skills.
- *Demonstration* and *return demonstration* are part of skill laboratory experiences. Faculty also have the opportunity to role model positive behaviors in all teaching settings. Listening, respecting others, asking questions, providing support, and seeking learners, input are constructive actions.

- *Learning contracts* between faculty and individual learners are useful for working on specialized projects. A contract requires learners to be self-directed. Adult learners can use their prior knowledge and expertise to develop new skills. When learners have different backgrounds, a contract allows them to progress at different rates and levels (Billings & Halstead, 2008).

FAST FACTS in a NUTSHELL

- Internally, budget constraints impact programs. Identify options to maintain quality as well as efficient programs.
- Externally, pay close attention to meeting standards, regulations, and guidelines.
- Include a variety of teaching strategies to meet the needs of diverse learners.

EXAMPLES OF COURSE DESIGNS

Carnegie Mellon University: Design and Teach Your Course

Many of the decisions affecting the success of a course take place well before the first day of class. Careful planning at the course design stage not only makes teaching easier and more enjoyable; it also facilitates student learning. Once your course is planned, teaching involves implementing your course design on a day-to-day level.

www.nursingcenter.com/library/JournalArticle.asp?Article_ID=818349

Lippincott Nursing Center: Designing and Delivering Effective Online Nursing Courses with the Evolve Electronic Classroom.

oct.sfsu.edu/design/content/htmls/design.html

San Francisco State University: Designing Course Content

www.ehow.com/how_6130013_create-using-addie-model-nursing.html

University of Phoenix: How to Create a Training Course Using ADDIE Model for Nursing

EXAMPLES OF TEACHING STRATEGIES

owl.english.purdue.edu/owl/resource/671/04/

Purdue University: Writing in nursing bibliography.

Provides an introduction to writing across the curriculum and writing in the disciplines, a list of links to WAC/WID programs, and a selected bibliography for further reading.

hsc.unm.edu/consg/critical/strategies.shtml

The University of New Mexico College of Nursing site explains a range of teaching strategies and includes video demonstrations.

PART

IV

Evaluation of Programs
and Curricula

13

Purposes and Examples of Program Outcomes

INTRODUCTION

Approval/accrediting agencies require nursing programs to identify outcomes that are achieved at the end of the program. In addition, many higher education institutions also require all programs, including nursing, to address the institution-wide general outcomes for all graduates. Nursing program outcomes are not the same as educational outcomes. Where educational outcomes specify what the learner is expected to demonstrate at completion of the nursing program, nursing program outcomes identify the expectations for all elements of a program.

In this chapter, you will learn:

1. The purpose of nursing program outcomes.
2. The essential parts of nursing program outcomes.

PURPOSE OF NURSING PROGRAM OUTCOMES

The purpose of nursing program outcomes is to guide data collection for periodic assessment of health program effectiveness. The results are analyzed and used to guide health program decisions.

===========================*FAST FACTS in a NUTSHELL*

- Nursing program outcomes are comprehensive and address all major areas: curriculum, faculty, learners, and resources.
- The outcomes provide information about the quality and effectiveness of a nursing program.

Definition of Key Terms
- A **nursing program outcome** is a measurable statement about what the nursing program expects to do or accomplish, a declarative and measurable statement assessing the effectiveness of the nursing program.

KEY POINTS

Do not confuse nursing program outcomes with educational, level, course, or individual learner outcomes. Educational and level outcomes are learning outcomes and address the learning that you want to occur. They are learner oriented.

Nursing program outcomes address the quality and effectiveness of the nursing program. They are nursing program oriented.

Nursing program outcomes are used to determine if the program mission is being met. Before identifying nursing program outcomes, a review of the nursing program mission statement should occur.

External approval/accrediting agencies require nursing program outcomes to address certain criteria, such as pass rates on licensing examinations, retention rates, learner/ employer satisfaction, job placement, etc.

External approval/accrediting agencies may designate the acceptable level for a particular nursing program outcome, such as the pass rate for first-time testers on the licensing examination shall be at least 80%. Approval/accrediting agencies usually include the required criteria in the nursing program evaluation standard.

In addition, many organization/parent institutions require nursing program outcomes to address identified general education attributes required for all graduates regardless of program, such as critical thinking, computer competency, communication, etc.

When developing nursing program outcomes, clearly state what will be assessed (e.g., licensure pass rates for first-time testers). Make sure the outcome is measurable. Identifying a realistic measurement process at this point in development is helpful. Make sure the outcome measures something useful and meaningful. The assessment approaches should produce evidence that is credible, suggestive, and applicable in order to make nursing program decisions.

Determine the acceptable level for success. Some success levels are determined by external agencies and others will be determined internally, by the organization/institution or the nursing program.

FAST FACTS in a NUTSHELL

- Nursing program outcomes focus on quality and effectiveness.
- All major aspects of a nursing program are evaluated.
- Specific measures must be determined.
- Outcomes must list the expected level of success.

Essential Elements of Outcome Statements

There are three major elements of outcomes statements (Table 13.1). Each outcome must have a specific focus so it can be measured. Grouping different areas together makes it difficult to measure specific outcomes. Once an area, such as

TABLE 13.1 Nursing Program Outcome Examples

Outcome Focus	Measurement	Measurement Target/ Standards
Retention	University registrar graduation report	80% of learners who begin the nursing program and who do not voluntarily withdraw will complete the four-year program within five years with a "C" or better.
RN Licensing Pass Rate	State board of nursing licensure NCLEX-RN® report by nursing program	80% of graduates from the nursing program will pass the NCLEX-RN on the first attempt.
Job Placement	Institution survey of graduates at 6 and 12 months after graduation	90% of graduates from the nursing program who actually seek employment will be employed in nursing 6 and 12 months after graduation.
Graduate Satisfaction with Nursing Program	Institution survey of graduates at 6 and 12 months after graduation	80% of the graduates will strongly agree or agree that the nursing program met stated outcomes.
Employer Satisfaction	Institution survey of graduates at 6 and 12 months after graduation	90% of employers will strongly agree or agree that the nursing program prepared the graduates for beginning level RN positions. The new RNs were able to practice nursing safely and competently.

(continued)

TABLE 13.1 Nursing Program Outcome Examples (*continued*)

Outcome Focus	Measurement	Measurement Target/ Standards
Communication (Organization/ Parent Institution Requirement)	Institution-required Capstone Research Project completed by the beginning of the last semester before graduation Oral presentation, based on institution guidelines, at the beginning of the last semester before graduation	90% of the graduates from the nursing program will demonstrate effective verbal and written communication skills by meeting the minimum requirements.
Critical Thinking (Organization/ Institution Requirement)	Nursing program-selected standardized critical thinking examination Institution-required Capstone Research Project completed by the beginning of the last semester before graduation	90% of graduates from the nursing program will demonstrate the ability to think critically by meeting the minimum requirements.

From S. B. Keating, 2006.

graduate satisfaction with the program, is determined, it is possible to use different measures to get more information. For example, having a survey to determine level of satisfaction is a good start. Collecting additional information from comments, phone interviews, or face-to-face sessions provides additional information—personal and memorable experiences, aspects of clinical experiences, or faculty creativity.

The second element is determining how to measure the outcomes. There are a wide variety of evaluation strategies, such as portfolio, simulation, role playing, essay, oral presentations, videotaping, and various types of examinations (Billings & Halsted, 2008). Select one or more methods that are appropriate for the outcome. Institutional documents and notes from nursing program meetings are also used to support the achievement of outcomes.

The third element is setting the minimal levels for successful achievement. The level may be stated numerically (quantitative) or descriptive (qualitative).

EXAMPLES OF NURSING PROGRAM OUTCOMES

While nursing program outcomes have common elements, they are individualized for each program based on internal and external requirements and expectations. The following are examples of the elements.

14

Purposes and Examples of Systematic Program Evaluation

INTRODUCTION

Systematic program evaluation planning begins when a program is first developed or revised. As the foundation of a nursing/health program is developed, it is essential to plot out the elements to evaluate.

Once all the program pieces are in place, it is essential to specify the elements for program evaluation. Data can then be collected in a systematic way at the beginning of the program.

Data collection is continuous. The steps of the process are carried out on a regular basis. One of the common deficiencies for programs, as they are reviewed, is lack of data about the effectiveness and quality of the education.

A major value of systematic evaluation is the ability to trend data over time: semester, year, or multiple years.

A systematic evaluation plan is the "big picture" of what is changing and includes the evidence about what was done to support effectiveness and quality.

In this chapter, you will learn:

1. The purposes of a systematic evaluation plan.
2. The essential parts of a systematic evaluation plan.

PURPOSES OF A SYSTEMATIC EVALUATION PLAN

Educational programs have been evaluated in different ways for many years. A traditional approach to evaluation of higher educational programs was to measure quality based on achievements of new students, faculty reputation, books and other learning resources, curricula, and student services. Essentially, the process consisted of counting the different areas.

Today, nursing and health educational programs are offered for diverse audiences in many different and sometimes nontraditional settings. Health education has become an essential part of nursing practice. Nurses teach patients and community groups in many different settings. This shift in teaching/learning requires looking at the outcomes of educational programs. The focus is on the end of an educational program—what do learners know and what are they able to do?

The reasons for this change are based on professional standards, guidelines, accreditation, and regulations from professional groups, accrediting agencies, and state/federal agencies. Evaluating outcomes provides information about learner achievement. It also helps the organizations offering health education programs to determine their effectives and make improvements.

A major accomplishment of the systematic evaluation approach is the ability to measure what learners actually gain from their educational programs. Systematic program evaluation plans provide the information, data, analysis, and decisions to ensure learners, educational institutions, and agencies have quality programs.

ESSENTIAL ELEMENTS OF SYSTEMATIC PROGRAM EVALUATION PLANS

Systematic evaluation is based on a very detailed plan. For educational programs, all the levels of evaluation are included with descriptions and examples of how all the elements flow from each other and are linked. The common elements of evaluation are listed in Table 14.1.

═══*FAST FACTS in a NUTSHELL*

- A nursing/health program is a subsystem of the institution/agency.
- A nursing/health program is interdependent within the institution/agency.
- A program must be a "fit" with the mission and philosophy of the institution/agency.
- Internal/external standards, regulations, and guidelines will influence nursing/health program evaluation.

TABLE 14.1 Essential Elements of a Systematic Program Evaluation Plan

Mission and governance of the institution/agency (mission, goals, purpose, and philosophy)

Institutional/organizational administration policies

Faculty/teachers

Learners

Curriculum and instruction

Resources

Outcomes/educational effectiveness

Learner academic achievement

Definition of Key Terms

- **Accrediting agencies** are professional groups that accredit institutions and nursing/health programs.
- **Assessment** means the processes used to systematically collect information to judge the value and significance related to program review and actions.
- **Benchmarking** is setting standards/criteria to measure educational program outcomes and to also compare results to other similar programs.
- **Continuous quality improvement** is when system processes carry out assessments and evaluate them regularly.
- **Evaluation** consists of analyzing results of data collected, sharing feedback, implementing recommendations, and repeating the processes on a schedule.
- **Goal** is a statement that is comprehensive, long term, and future focused.
- **Objective** is a description of performance, condition, and criteria related to behaviors that indicate a level of learning.
- **Outcome evaluation** is when program goals are connected to outcome objectives and provide comprehensive evaluation at the end of a program.
- **Regulatory agencies** are government groups that approve, monitor, and evaluate institutions and programs.
- **Required standards** are standards developed by governmental and regulatory agencies, professional accrediting bodies, and specialized standards that focus on specific areas such as distance education.

================================*FAST FACTS in a NUTSHELL*

- Develop a list of terms that are specific to your institution/agency so everyone has a common understanding.
- Understand what terms used in standards, regulations, and guidelines mean.
- Consistently use the same terms when discussing and presenting assessment and evaluation data.

KEY POINTS

Determine the Persons in an Institution/Agency Responsible for Developing a Plan

When a program is being developed or revised, a committee or group should be selected. Nurses have many commitments and may be overwhelmed by their usual workload and may not want to participate. It is essential that there is broad representation because of the different types of information that are collected. Administrative support, in terms of financial resources, released time, staff, and technology requirements, is needed to develop, revise, and sustain data collection and analysis.

Select the standards or guidelines that are required for the program to determine the essential elements of the plan. That information provides a foundation to develop the specific areas for assessment and evaluation.

Designating one person to be "in charge" and providing staff support should ensure that the schedule is maintained. There are computer-based project planning programs that can identify the smallest tasks with who should complete them and when. These can be updated for all participants to see the progress.

Timeline to Develop and Implement a Plan

A common problem is not allowing enough time to develop and implement a plan. It is useful to look at the desired end result. When would an external review or accreditation visit be scheduled? When would documentation have to be submitted? If writing a grant, when is the submission date? Internally, what are the deadlines for submitting budget requests? How many levels of approval are required for the plan?

These factors need to be included in the planning process. There can be a "fast track" for developing or revising a plan if there is an existing model or some elements, such as a budget, have been preapproved.

Once a timeline is drafted, add weeks/months to the major elements, if possible. It is better to finish early than to miss deadlines.

═══════════════════════════════*FAST FACTS in a NUTSHELL*

- Include broad participation to have the expertise and number of persons needed.
- Consider a wide range of internal and external factors that will impact the timeline for the development/revision of the plan.

Evaluation Methods

Because there are so many different elements in program evaluation, there are many different approaches used to collect and analyze the information.

The method(s) selected must be consistent over time to ensure the data can be trended. If one method is used in Year 1 of data collection, and another method is used in Year 2, it will be difficult or impossible to trend data for multiple years. Nursing faculty and administrators need to assess the elements for a set period of time and only make changes when there are problems or changes in outcomes.

Program methods may include questionnaires, interviews, observation, rating scales, checklists, attitude scales, self-report journals, informal notes, and records of conferences and meetings (Billings & Halstead, 2008).

It is useful to use multiple methods to gain a comprehensive picture of what learners can actually do. Because there are so many possibilities, the methods selected must clearly measure the outcomes. Methods may include demonstration of skills, case methods to solve problems, presentations, and written papers.

Determine Actions:
Development, Maintenance, or Revision

The results of a systematic evaluation plan can be divided into three categories:

Development; additional teaching/learning strategies, use of new technology, and new policies to meet changes in internal and/or external requirements.
Maintenance; no changes for elements that met or exceeded benchmarks, and no reason to make a change unless there are new strategies to further improve or internal and external requirements.
Revisions; based on new evidence of best practices, successful strategies used in other program, or additional internal and external requirements

Approaches to Reporting Evaluation Outcomes

Reports developed to present the program outcome information should include the following basic areas (Western Washington University, 2011):

    What did you do?
    Why did you do it?
    What did you find?
    How will you use it?
    What is your evaluation of the assessment plan itself?
    Did it include all the essential elements?

All systematic evaluation plans yield a great deal of information that is used in different ways. The purpose of a report and the intended audience is considered. External reviewers will have a set way they expect the data to be organized and reported. Within the institution/agency, summary information is useful for executive reports. Public announcements will highlight what is important for those audiences.

FAST FACTS in a NUTSHELL

- Select multiple evaluation methods and consistently collect data for meaningful results over time.
- Determine if results support development, maintenance, or revision and make appropriate decisions to improve the program.
- Adapt the reporting of outcomes to meet the needs of different audiences.

EXAMPLES OF SYSTEMATIC EVALUATION PLANS

While systematic evaluation plans have common elements, they are individualized for each program based on internal and external requirements and expectations. Table 14.2 shows examples of the elements.

TABLE 14.2 Examples of Essential Elements of a Systematic Program Evaluation Plan

Mission and governance of the institution/agency (mission, goals, purpose, and philosophy)	• Documentation of faculty consensus with institutional and program mission and philosophy.
Institutional/ organizational administration policies	• Review of committee and other documents for evidence of faculty governance in the institution.
Faculty/teachers/learners	• Summary profile of program faculty compared to all faculty in an institution (qualifications, professional development, service, and scholarship accomplishments). • Results of standardized tests and licensure/certification outcomes related to other similar programs.

(continued)

TABLE 14.2 Examples of Essential Elements of a Systematic Program Evaluation Plan (*continued*)	
Curriculum and instruction	• Program faculty report describes current status of curriculum and how the outcome results support the need for improvement in certain areas.
Resources	• Outcomes that have not achieved identified goals can be used to gain additional resources (faculty, equipment, etc.) in the next budget cycle.
Outcomes/educational effectiveness	• Data from questionnaires, interviews, observation, rating scales, checklists, attitude scales, self-report journals, informal notes, and records of conferences and meetings (Billings & Halstead, 2008).
Learner academic achievement	• A process will be **developed** to include the new requirement for a program exit standardized exam that is required for graduation. • The licensing examination pass rate is at 97%, which is 10% above the national average. That rate will be **maintained** for the program. • The attrition rate for the program is 10% higher than the institution and national standards. The data will be reviewed and **revisions** implemented to reduce the rate to equal the standards.

15

Purposes and Examples
of Systematic Data Collection

INTRODUCTION

Many approval/accrediting agencies require nursing programs to collect data for program outcomes. In addition, many higher education institutions also require data from all programs to address the institution-wide general outcomes for all graduates. Nursing program outcomes identify the end-of-program expectations and are usually reported as aggregate data.

In this chapter, you will learn:

1. Outcomes give details of what was accomplished and relates them to mission, regulations, and standards.
2. To develop outcomes to assess end-of-program accomplishments.
3. To organize and share the summarized data.
4. To use data to make improvements in programs.

PURPOSES OF NURSING PROGRAM SYESTEMATIC DATA COLLECTION

Data are collected for the entire program to look at the "big picture." The data are examined to see how all the curriculum and assessment/evaluation pieces fit together. Analysis of outcome data can answer the following questions:

To what extent do program outcomes support the mission, goals, and desired organizational outcomes?
Was the program implemented as planned?
Were the different types of resources used efficiently?
What are program strengths and what improvements are needed?
Do the data justify decisions made to improve the educational offering?

It is essential to trend data for a period of time, three to five years, to evaluate changes in program outcomes and make significant changes if indicated. Making changes based on only one year of data may not indicate what is really happening within the program (Billings & Halstead, 2008). The purposes can be applied to any type of educational program.

============================*FAST FACTS in a NUTSHELL*

- Collect data that presents the "big picture" of the program.
- Collect the same data over three to five years to trend changes.
- Use data to make decisions about program changes.

Definition of Key Terms

- **Aggregated data** are evaluation information that is organized and summarized from specific evaluation sources so that it can be viewed as a whole.
- **Benchmarks** are specific standards or criteria used by educational institutions or organizations to measure program success and to make comparisons with similar programs (Billings & Halstead, 2008).
- **Development actions based on outcome data** are the addition of new teaching, learning, or evaluation strategies to improve programs.
- **Executive summary** is a brief document that summarizes the key points of a longer report. Using the same headings and referring, by page numbers, to the original documents allows the reader to look at more information if desired. Often created for busy executives who do not have the time to read long reports.
- **Maintenance actions based on outcome data** are the continuation of actions without revisions/changes because the outcomes were met.
- **Nursing program outcomes** comprise a measurable statement about what the nursing program expects to do or accomplish, a declarative and measurable statement assessing the effectiveness of the nursing program.
- **Program assessment** consists of processes to gather information about all aspects of a program to determine if standards and benchmarks are met.
- **Qualitative data** are information collected from verbal, written, or other formats that do not include numbers.
- **Quantitative data** are information collected in numeric (number) formats.
- **Revision actions based on outcome data** are changes/improvements made to current teaching, learning, and assessment strategies to improve programs.

• **Stakeholders** are internal and external individuals and groups who have an interest and responsibility for program quality and effectiveness. Examples include administrators, accrediting and approval agencies, funding agencies, employers, and graduates.

KEY POINTS

• Program outcomes focus on all aspects: curriculum, resources, faculty, environment, students, and services.
• Program outcome assessment is comprehensive and usually done on an annual basis.
• Select assessment methods that are congruent with the outcomes (simple to complex) and the available resources (low to high technology).
• Use multiple types of assessments to include cognitive, affective, and psychomotor domains as appropriate.
• Have a system in place to efficiently and effectively carry out evaluation activities.
• Consistently use the same methods for three to five years to be able to trend program outcomes.
• When changes in data collection are needed, justify the rationale (new standards, new technologies, organizational requirements, and inadequacy of a current method).
• Sharing outcomes, with stakeholders, is an essential step in the evaluation process to continue program improvement.

═══════════════════════════*FAST FACTS in a NUTSHELL*

• Collect data for all major areas of the program.
• Determine a schedule for data analysis that fits with required internal and external reports.
• Use data to justify and support decisions about program changes.

EXAMPLES OF NURSING PROGRAM DATA COLLECTION

Standardized Test Scores Compared to State and National Outcomes

Nursing students take standardized tests during and at the end of their programs to assess their readiness to pass the licensing exam for their profession. Results of standardized assessments provide both learners and teachers with detailed information about strengths and weaknesses. Teachers can make appropriate revisions to course content when weaknesses are aggregated for specific areas. Learners have individual results and can focus on their weak areas so they are prepared for their licensing exam.

State boards of nursing and regulatory agencies for other health-related programs have specific levels of performance required to maintain approval.

In one nursing program, the pass rate on the licensing exam for the previous academic year was 85%. The pass rate has been between 85% and 87% for the past three years. The national average for the current year was 94% and the average for the three previous years was 93%. The state board of nursing required a minimum of an 85% pass rate for continued approval.

The faculty were committed to having a higher pass rate that matched the national rate. The current benchmark is 85%, which means that the outcome has been met. The goal was to set the benchmark at 90% for the next two years, with the option to raise it when the 90% outcome is met for at least two years.

The school of nursing program evaluation and assessment committee reviewed student outcomes for all the categories and subcategories on the licensing exam and also the standardized course exam outcomes in the same categories to see if there are similar weak areas. Faculty will review and revise weak specific content in cognitive, affective, and psychomotor domains.

Survey Results From External Stakeholders and Graduates

Nursing programs need to collect data from clinical agencies to determine how well the students and graduates were prepared for clinical experiences and their first positions after graduation. Surveys are commonly used. It is important to use methods that do not take a great deal of time, ask questions directly related to program outcomes, and allow for both qualitative and quantitative data.

The actual data collection can be done electronically by sending surveys to the stakeholders and having them returned the same way. Technology services can aggregate the data according to your specifications. Quantitative data are collected this way, with options for additional comments for qualitative data.

Another option is face-to-face or telephone sessions with focused questions. This method primarily collects qualitative data. Using at least two methods provides a range of data.

EXAMPLES OF AN ORGANIZATION/AGENCY SYSTEMATIC DATA COLLECTION

A diabetic education program has six modules. They were developed for learners to progress on a continuum of knowledge about their condition to self management. Within each module, the content moves from simple to complex.

A review could include looking at learner responses about the organization of the program.

Assessment of learner satisfaction outcome: The desired outcome was to determine learners' satisfaction with the organization of the program. The benchmark was that 85% of the learners who completed the program would be satisfied or highly satisfied with the course.

There were a total of 200 learners who completed the program in the past twelve months. One hundred forty-five (72.50%) responded to the survey with four choices: highly satisfied, satisfied, somewhat satisfied, and not satisfied. One hundred thirty (89%) were satisfied/highly satisfied.

The teachers reviewed the data and determined they would maintain what they were doing but would also look at all the somewhat and not satisfied responses to determine if there were patterns in those responses that indicated revisions were needed.

The organizational mission and goals were compared to the program outcomes. If the organization has a mission to meet the needs of diverse groups, then the learners should have those characteristics. If the program was presented only in English and the diverse groups in the community use different languages, then changes and improvements are needed. Additional stakeholders may need to be added to the program planning process.

Assessment of learner diversity in program: The desired outcome is that the program learners reflect the cultural and language diversity of the local population with diabetes.

Current census and the public health department data indicate that of the population over 50 years of age, 20% are Hispanic, 10% are Asian, 20% are African American, and 40% are Caucasian. The remainder of the population is "other."

The classes offered during the previous years had a similar distribution of learners, except for the Hispanic (6%) and African American (5%) groups.

A 2007–2009 national survey of people diagnosed with diabetes, aged 20 years or older, included the following prevalence by race/ethnicity (http://www.diabetes.org American Diabetes Association):

7.1% of non-Hispanic Whites
8.4% of Asian Americans
12.6% of non-Hispanic Blacks
11.8% of Hispanics

The teachers developed a plan to invite members of Hispanic and African American ethnic organizations to get input about attracting more persons to the classes.

The organization uses computer technology in all areas of its operations. The diabetic education program was developed from this perspective. During implementation it became apparent that participants needed extensive training, and some became discouraged and dropped out. The teachers knew changes were needed in this area. Other low-technology options should be developed and used.

The teachers kept informal notes from learners who did not complete the program. There were 50 who had dropped out of the program during the last year. Twenty-five mentioned they use a computer. The teachers planned to offer information in print form and would ask learners, when they signed up for the program, about their preferences.

Every organization is concerned about how their resources are used. Attendance records could show the number of learners at each session. That data could be used to decide if multiple sessions could be collapsed or new sections added. The number of staff at each session could be compared to the number of participants. The days, times, and locations of the education program can also be reviewed to determine if the resources were congruent with the needs.

The teachers reviewed the attendance and informal notes from learners about scheduling. Each session had a teacher/learner ratio of 1:10. This ratio was selected because learners could get individual attention, have their questions answered, and had 1:1 supervised skill demonstrations.

Learners who completed the program were asking for a support group to share information and get ideas maintain their healthy practices. The teachers developed a plan to have one session a month, to start, based on the most popular times the learners attend the programs. A diabetic nurse specialist would be responsible for the group and the hospital would provide space. A process for evaluating the support group was developed and would be implemented six months after the start of the group.

Look at all the data for the diabetic education program and compare it to the different benchmarks. Also, summarize the positive outcomes and prioritize the areas needing improvement. Determine if any new initiatives are needed. A concise presentation of the outcomes provides a holistic, readable document. Stakeholders and decision makers know what happened. Sharing the information in the media brings positive attention to the organization, increases interest, and provides possible opportunities for additional support (Anema & McCoy, 2010).

The previous examples propose different ways to assess program elements. Programs will have additional assessment elements based on organizational requirements, best practices mandated by professional groups, and governmental regulations.

When there are data on all the different elements, a total report should include all the information in summary form. It is essential to keep all the individual information from surveys, assessments, participation, and any other documents that were used to summarize the outcomes.

The result of the comprehensive outcome assessment needs to be widely shared. Different audiences and stakeholders need the information that is required and of interest to them.

Sharing the outcomes provides the administration with data to determine the value of the program, cost-benefit of the program, impact on hospitalization, evidence that quality standards were achieved, and decisions for making changes.

Marketing the diabetic education program and the addition of a support group makes the community aware of what the organization is doing for them.

Participants can agree to share their stories in the media.

Teachers and organizational representatives can appear in local public interest media and before community groups to share the information.

The program can receive awards for excellence and seek grant and other types of support for the program.

Expansion of the program could include younger age groups and presentation of educational programs in schools.

When organizations have quality programs that meet the needs of many persons in a community, it is very positive to share results with wide audiences. This aspect is often overlooked and the outcomes stay in the reports.

FAST FACTS in a NUTSHELL

- Individualize the types of data collected for a program.
- Compare collected data to benchmarks and external standards/guidelines.
- Consider using data to highlight achievements in the program.

SHARING SYSTEMATIC DATA COLLECTION

Nursing Program Outcome Data

External stakeholders need summarized reports related to specific areas. Leaders in the clinical sites are interested in summarized responses from the staff who worked with new graduates of the program. The survey would include how prepared the graduates were for practice. Student surveys of their clinical experiences at all the sites help the organization make improvements in students' experiences. Summarized reports for each agency should be developed and include qualitative responses as appropriate. Agencies can have an end of rotation or academic year meeting with faculty to discuss the students' experiences from their perspectives.

Pass rates and accreditation status are very important to clinical agencies. It is also useful to highlight how the improvements over the previous year made a positive difference for learner clinical skills. Survey data from the clinical agencies are included.

The evaluation and assessment committee will review student outcomes for all the categories and subcategories on the licensing exam and also the standardized exam outcomes in the same categories to see if there are similar weak areas.

Faculty will review that information and revise weak specific content or psychomotor skills areas.

Administrators and leaders need to see the big picture and have access to all the data. It is helpful to have a report or executive summary to share how specific outcomes met both the program and the organizational benchmarks.

An executive summary shares essential pieces of information with the university leaders. For example, the university goals of attrition, diversity of the student body, and scores on the university exit exam are included. The outcome areas were placed under each of the university goals. The information indicated university goal and benchmark, school of nursing outcomes were met. A comment may be added about the level of achievement.

Diabetic Education Program Outcome Data

Sharing outcomes provides the administration with data to determine the value of the program, cost-benefit of the program, impact on hospitalization, evidence that quality standards were achieved, and decisions for making changes.

Marketing the diabetic education program and the addition of a support group makes the community aware of what the organization is doing for them.

Participants can agree to share their stories in the media. Teachers and organizational representatives can appear in local public interest media and before community groups to share the information. The program can receive awards for excellence and seek grant and other types of support for the program. Expansion of the program could include younger age groups and presentation of educational programs in schools.

When organizations have quality programs that meet the needs of many persons in a community, it is very positive to share results with wide audiences. This aspect is often overlooked and the outcomes stay in the reports.

Look at all the data for the diabetic education program and compare it to the different benchmarks. Also, summarize the positive outcomes and prioritize the areas needing improvement. Determine if any new initiatives are needed. A concise presentation of the outcomes provides a holistic, readable document. Stakeholders and decision makers know what happened. Sharing the information in the media brings positive attention to the organization, increases interest, and provides possible opportunities for additional support (Anema & McCoy, 2010).

The previous examples propose different ways to collect outcome data for specific program elements. Programs will have additional assessment elements based on organizational requirements, best practices mandated by professional groups, and governmental regulations. When there are data on all the different elements, a total report should include all the information in summary form.

It is essential to keep all the individual information from surveys, assessments, participation, and any other documents that were used to summarize the outcomes.

The result of the comprehensive outcome assessment needs to be widely shared.

Different audiences and stakeholders need the information that is required and of interest to them.

═══════════════════════════════*FAST FACTS in a NUTSHELL*

- Determine which internal and external stakeholders need outcome data.
- Select a variety of approaches to share outcome data, based on different stakeholders.
- Provide outcome data in readable formats, based on stakeholders' need for specific types of information.

16

Purposes and Examples of Curriculum Data Collection

INTRODUCTION

Chapter 13 addressed program outcomes. This chapter focuses on assessing the learning that has taken place in individual courses. It is vital for learners and faculty to have evidence of each learner's achievement as well as overall course outcomes. Course improvements cannot be made by just reviewing individual results.

Combining or aggregating individual outcome data provides the "big picture" of what is happening in a course. Each course has criteria for assessing learning outcomes. The outcomes give details of what was accomplished and relates them to program and organizational benchmarks.

In this chapter, you will learn:

1. The purposes for collecting curriculum data.
2. The types of curriculum data to collect.
3. Strategies to organize the collected curriculum data.

PURPOSES OF CURRICULUM
DATA COLLECTION

There are several purposes for collecting data from each course in a curriculum. Data collection makes it possible to review the entire educational offering (curriculum/course) to determine how the pieces fit together. Data can be trended for a period of time, three to five years, to evaluate changes in learner outcomes and make significant changes if indicated. It is an opportunity to examine how the course outcomes support the mission, goals, and desired organizational outcomes. Collecting data provides information about how the educational offering was implemented as planned and to assess if the different types of resources were used efficiently. Data are also evaluated to determine course strengths and need for improvements.

=== *FAST FACTS in a NUTSHELL*

- Collect a variety of data to ensure all essential curriculum data are pulled together.
- Collect the same data for three to five years to trend course outcomes.
- Data needs to support program and institutional foundational documents.

Definition of Key Terms
- **Course assessments** gather information about learner learning outcomes.
- An **educational offering** is a collection/group of topics that are organized into a structured format.
- **Reliability of assessment measures** provide data that are dependable, precise, and consistent each time the measures are used (Billings & Halstead, 2008).

- **Rubrics** are specific statements that indicate what elements are found in assessments and their assigned values.
- **Qualitative data** are information collected from verbal, written, or other formats that do not include numbers.
- **Quantitative data** are information collected in numeric (number) formats.
- **Standard templates** are guides to help consistently evaluate assessments.
- **Learner learning outcomes** include the knowledge, attitudes, and skills learners demonstrate at the end of learning activities.
- **Validity of assessment measures** relates specifically to the program or course and provide meaningful data that support continuous improvement (Billings & Halstead, 2008).
- A **taxonomy** is a system for classifying groups or collections in order from low to high.

KEY POINTS

Courses focus on learner outcomes for selected content in a set timeframe. Look at both individual and course outcomes to determine if the outcomes were met. Learner learning outcomes (objectives) are the key to developing reliable and valid assessments that measure what is intended. Learning outcomes have different levels and are selected based on the desired knowledge and skills required.

Select assessment methods that are congruent with the outcomes (simple to complex) and the available resources (low to high technology). Use multiple types of assessments to include cognitive, affective, and psychomotor domains as appropriate. Bloom (1956) developed a taxonomy to select appropriate learner outcomes for different types of course outcomes. There are three domains (types) of learner outcomes: cognitive, affective, and psychomotor. Cognitive domains address the acquisition, integration, and application of knowledge. Affective domains address transformation of ideas, values, and feelings. Psychomotor domains address the acquisition of motor or physical skills. Within each domain, there are different levels.

The first few categories in each domain are appropriate expectations for beginning learner outcomes. Learners must initially have some information and understanding about the topics and content. As learners progress in their programs, they need to demonstrate more complex behaviors in each domain. Because nursing is a practice discipline, high levels of critical thinking, clinical skills, and professional behaviors are expected of graduates.

FAST FACTS in a NUTSHELL

- Collect data from three different domains: cognitive, affective, and psychomotor.
- Domains have levels, with the first categories for beginning learners.
- Collecting critical thinking, clinical skills, and professional behavior data is essential to determine graduates can provide safe, quality nursing care.

There are many types of assessments used to collect curriculum data. Some examples are:

- Unit examinations
- Comprehensive final examinations
- Standardized examinations
- Patient care plans
- Skill check-off forms
- Patient clinical class presentation
- Comprehensive course content formal paper

The value (grade) assigned to each assessment is based on the level, goals, and focus of each course. For example, beginning nursing courses will have multiple skills assessments and graduate-level nursing courses will focus on higher-level assessments such as research papers.

Other types of curriculum data that are collected are based on learner input and review course structures and processes. Some examples are:

- Standard templates to compare course learning outcomes with content and learner activities
- Standard templates to compare textbooks and course materials for currency of information
- Learner satisfaction surveys with classroom environment, teaching strategies, and teacher characteristics
- Written peer evaluations of learner presentations

FAST FACTS in a NUTSHELL

- Examinations, skills check-off lists, and care plans are commonly used to collect data.
- Values (points/grades) are determined by course levels and types of assessments.
- Collecting information from the learners is an important data source.

Data are collected in two main formats: quantitative and qualitative. The majority of data are collected in a numerical/number format. Scores on exams, points for written assignments, and percentages for correct answers are examples of quantitative data. Qualitative data do not have numbers and are found in survey responses, verbal responses to questions, and self-reflection about experiences and learning. Choices may be from poor to excellent or from disagree to agree or general comments about thoughts and feelings. Numeric values are added to responses. For example, 50% of the learners who responded to the survey agreed the course presentations were excellent.

Once the assessments are completed, data analysis and rubrics are used to determine scores and grades. Validity refers to the appropriateness and usefulness of the data related to the identified curriculum outcomes. Review the content of the assessments to assure it includes the essential evaluation elements. Reliability refers to the ability of an assessment to demonstrate consistent results each time the data are collected (Billings & Halstead, 2008).

Have a system in place to efficiently and effectively carry out assessment activities.

Collecting quantitative data is usually done using some type of technology. Learners may take examinations on a computer and software compiles the results for each learner and also aggregates it for the course. Learners may fill out scanning forms, which are also graded electronically. Survey forms can be done on a computer and the results analyzed. Using technology is very helpful for large groups and when data are collected on a regular schedule. It also is efficient and eliminates human error.

Qualitative data may also be collected using technology for surveys, which can include space for individual comments. It is more challenging to review written assignments and then collect data that identify problem areas. Specific grading rubrics help focus the grading decisions. If technology is not available, using paper and pencil forms for data collection is an option.

Oral data may be collected using recordings and notes from group sessions. Two or more people can review the information for consistency and accuracy.

============================*FAST FACTS in a NUTSHELL*

- The majority of curriculum data are collected with numerical (quantitative) information.
- Qualitative data (non-numerical) add curriculum outcome data from different perspectives: opinions, reflections, and suggestions for improvement.

EXAMPLES OF CURRICULUM DATA COLLECTION

Learning outcomes have different levels and are selected based on the desired knowledge and skills required. In nursing education, there is an emphasis on collecting data in the following areas.

Comprehension Examples

- Describe the steps to self-administer insulin.
- Explain two ways to take temperatures.

Application Examples

- Apply the principles of sterile technique to opening a sterile kit.
- Calculate the IV infusion rate from the information given: gtts per minute, type of fluid, and IV tubing.

Analysis Examples

- Interpret the laboratory results to make a decision about potential care actions.
- Differentiate between primary and secondary care decisions.

Synthesis Examples

- Design a comprehensive care plan for a new client.
- Update the process for informing patients of their privacy rights, based on new federal guidelines.

Evaluation Examples

- Rank three treatment approaches for their effectiveness in resolving foot ulcers.
- Justify the purchase of new oxygen therapy equipment.

Examples of Assessment Methods

- At the end of a class on self-administration of insulin, learners complete a written test and demonstrate doing a skills task in person or on a video tape.
- Alumni surveys use fill-in, open-ended questions that are completed online or in small group sessions.
- Written learner satisfaction with classroom environment, teaching strategies, and teacher characteristics are done online or with paper surveys.
- Written peer evaluations are provided of learner presentations.

Examples of Organizing Curriculum Data Collection

A faculty evaluation and assessment committee is conducting a comprehensive review for all the course outcomes.

- A university computer center stores most of the outcome assessment data. Teachers have access to a report with individual scores and the item analysis of each question. They also receive summarized data for their course evaluations. Learner names are not shown on the results but the number of responses on the scale is listed.

- Additionally, the software program can read comments and insert them in the course evaluation summary.
- Teachers track individual trends in their courses and use the outcome information as part of their annual performance review.
- The information is kept on the server and different reports are generated when requested. Individuals and the program can print out any report they want for their own files.
- Individual courses are assessed each time they are completed.
- Individual learner results, from exams and other assignments, are available so both learners and teachers can review the results.
- Surveys, teacher evaluations, learner services, and organizational characteristics are grouped and anonymous.
- Teachers also receive reports after each exam. Reports list individual learner results as well as highest and lowest scores, median, mean, item discrimination, item difficulty, standard deviation, test reliability, and standard error of measurement.
- There is software to help organize qualitative data, but the essence of it may be lost. Original comments from learners, employees, and anyone who receives or provides services can be used for several purposes.
- Faculty need results of individual assessments in addition to the aggregated data for examinations, with common statistics.

FAST FACTS in a NUTSHELL

- Include different domain levels (comprehension, application, analysis, synthesis, and evaluation) in data collection.
- Technology and software are available to organize all types of quantitative data.
- Qualitative data are often organized by summarizing the main points.
- Curriculum data collection is needed by learners to know their progress and by faculty to examine outcomes.

17

Using Outcome Data to Support Quality Nursing Education

INTRODUCTION

Outcome program and course data are collected for analysis and review with a goal of improving a program. The data are aggregated using appropriate statistical methods to determine if learners achieved the expected benchmark outcomes in a course. Program outcome data goes beyond individual courses and includes faculty, environmental, financial, institutional support, clinical facilities, and other elements that are part of quality education. Faculty need to recognize how all the program elements affect the quality of a program. It is also essential that internal and external stakeholders have the information in formats that make it easy to interpret the data correctly and can use it to make decisions.

In this chapter, you will learn:

1. To evaluate outcome data for use in program improvement.
2. To relate outcome data to program benchmarks.

3. To use outcome data to make improvements in programs.
4. To select approaches to share outcome data with students, faculty, and other internal and external stakeholders.

PURPOSES OF USING CURRICULUM OUTCOME DATA

Before there was a focus on outcomes for all types of educational programs, the focus was on the processes related to teaching and learning. A major accomplishment of the assessment movement is a focus on important questions about what students actually gain from their experiences at colleges and universities. Institutions are now held accountable to evaluate teaching, learning, and other processes for program outcomes. A major purpose for using the data from systematic program evaluation is to ensure students, the public, and employers that educational institutions provide quality and value. Another purpose is to have support for decisions made to add new program options, meet new standards, or improve existing ones. Trending outcomes over time helps decision-makers change what they are doing. All the purposes are connected to assuring graduates are prepared for nursing practice.

====================================*FAST FACTS in a NUTSHELL*

- Organize data according to identified outcomes.
- Assess trended data and summarize how it has changed.
- Categorize data according to actions: development, maintenance, or revision.

Definition of Key Terms
- **Aggregate data** are combined information and their analysis, using statistical and other methods to see group outcomes.

KEY POINTS

Deciding how to use and present the data starts with matching it with each of the program and course outcome data. For example, if an outcome is that all faculty will have master's degrees in nursing and specialization in the area they teach, create a table that lists their credentials and the courses/clinical they are teaching. A format may be developed from previous accreditation visits and it can be updated. If course data show that learners consistently did poorly in drug calculations, look at the specific areas, review teaching learning strategies, and identify the available resources.

Once all the data are reviewed, the actions fall into three general categories:

- **Development** of new teaching/learning strategies, use of new technology, and new policies to meet changes in internal and/or external requirements.
- **Maintenance** of elements that have met or exceeded benchmarks. There is no reason to make a change unless there are new strategies to further improve or meet new internal and external requirements.
- **Revisions** are done when content information is updated because of new evidence and standards. Learner input regarding examinations, the teaching learning environment, and clinical experiences can support revisions. Additionally, the data may support revisions in the way processes are done and policies are implemented.

In many situations, faculty spend a great deal of time reviewing what they are teaching and make changes that are not based on data. The process of working on curriculum and courses can be part of a culture where individual preferences are followed. Changes in faculty also contribute to this activity. It is one that many faculty feel comfortable with and enjoy doing. The issue is that data are not used for the changes and may not make a difference in the outcomes. For example, if a class complains that the examinations are too difficult or there are too many of them, faculty may make changes based on that information. The result of this approach is there is not evidence that changes are based on outcome data. The question of why and how the decisions were made cannot be answered with any support or justification.

Developing a plan to specify what changes are needed and how they will be done is essential. Course changes are proposed by the faculty teaching in those areas and submitted to the curriculum committee. Policy and procedure changes are discussed by the entire faculty, approved, and submitted to the program administrators. Changes that relate to institution/organization policies and procedures are approved in the nursing program and moved forward to the higher levels. Depending on the type of changes, there are guidelines for implementation. For example, if a course is added to the program, it will be implemented when new learners start.

Benchmarks are guides for setting the minimum levels of performance for both course and program outcomes. They clearly identify what are acceptable outcomes. Table 17.1 provides examples.

Evidence of best practices and success from other programs provides a foundation for making decisions. Review current literature, talk with colleagues, and attend professional meetings. Outcome data provide support for why changes are needed. The next question is, how should it be done? If there is a critical problem, such as the NCLEX-RN® pass rate, then a review of the total curriculum content to determine what is taught and to see if the essential elements are reinforced along with remediation and additional practice time is a priority. The weak areas on the practice exam and NCLEX-RN results reports will focus decisions. Other decisions, based on the outcomes data, may be less critical. If writing skills do not meet the benchmark values, then a more comprehensive plan to address this at all levels, both within the program

TABLE 17.1 BSN Nursing Program Benchmarks

Benchmarks	Nursing Outcomes
Clinical Practice Competency	95% of learners will demonstrate competency in their clinical experiences at the completion of each course as evidenced by the term grade reports.
End-of-Program NCLEX-RN Practice Examination	90% of learners will earn passing grades on the NCLEX-RN practice test the first time they take the course as evidenced by the testing service report.
Senior Capstone Project	95% of learners will satisfactorily complete the senior capstone project as evidenced by the term grade reports.
Program Retention	85% of learners, who begin the BSN program and who do not voluntarily withdraw, will complete the nursing program within three years with grades of "C" or better in the nursing courses as evidenced by registrar graduation report.
NCLEX-RN Pass Rate	90% of graduates from the BSN program will pass the NCLEX-RN on the first attempt as evidenced by state board of nursing licensure report.
Job Placement	95% of graduates from the BSN program who actually seek employment will be employed in nursing 6 to 9 months after graduation as evidenced by six-month survey results.
Learner Satisfaction	95% of the graduates of the BSN program will strongly agree or agree that the program met stated outcomes as evidenced by six-month survey results.
Employer Satisfaction	95% of employers strongly agree or agree that they are satisfied with the BSN program graduates' ability to practice nursing safely and competently as evidenced by six-month survey results.
Communication (Organization/ Parent Institution Requirement)	100% of the graduates from the BSN program will demonstrate effective verbal and written communication skills as evidenced by the Capstone Project.
Critical Thinking (Organization/ Parent Institution Requirement)	100% of graduates from the BSN program will demonstrate the ability to think critically as evidenced by the critical thinking examination.

and the liberal arts courses, can be developed. Faculty discuss possibilities and need to include financial, human, and other resources. Administrators need to approve new options and find the resources.

Trending data over a period of time makes it possible to see if and how the outcomes are making a positive difference or are maintaining the course and program elements. Simple tables can be used to display aggregated outcome data by year as it is collected. This format is used in reports. Software programs are used to collect and aggregate it. Table 17.2 provides examples.

TABLE 17.2 BSN Nursing Program Trending Data

Nursing Program Outcome 1

85% of learners, who begin the BSN program and who do not voluntarily withdraw, will complete the nursing program within three years with grades of "C" or better in the nursing courses as evidenced by registrar graduation report.

Year	Class of 2011	Class of 2012	Class of 2013	Class of 2014	Class of 2015
No. admitted					
No. completed					
Completion %					

Five-year aggregate =

Nursing Program Outcome 2

90% of graduates from the BSN program will pass the NCLEX-RN on the first attempt as evidenced by state board of nursing licensure report.

Year	Class of 2011	Class of 2012	Class of 2013	Class of 2014	Class of 2015
No. of first attempt pass					
% of first attempt pass					

Five-year aggregate =

(continued)

TABLE 17.2 BSN Nursing Program Trending Data (*continued*)

Nursing Program Outcome 3

95% of graduates from the BSN program who actually seek employment will be employed in nursing 6 to 9 months after graduation as evidenced by six-month survey results.

Year	Class of 2011	Class of 2012	Class of 2013	Class of 2014	Class of 2015
No. employed					
Employment %					

Five-year aggregate =

Nursing Program Outcome 4

95% of the graduates of the BSN program will strongly agree or agree that the program met stated outcomes as evidenced by six-month survey results.

Year	Class of 2011	Class of 2012	Class of 2013	Class of 2014	Class of 2015
No. strongly agree or agree					
Strongly agree or agree %					

Five-year aggregate =

Nursing Program Outcome 5

95% of employers strongly agree or agree that they are satisfied with the BSN program graduates' ability to practice nursing safely and competently as evidenced by six-month survey results.

Year	Class of 2011	Class of 2012	Class of 2013	Class of 2014	Class of 2015
No. strongly agree or agree					
Strongly agree or agree %					

Five-year aggregate =

TABLE 17.3 Setting Up Data Collection Process

BSN Outcome	Time	Discussion	Action
Critical thinking	Fall 2008	A standardized test subscale was used to evaluate critical thinking. Benchmark was set that 90% of learners would achieve at least 75%.	Benchmark was met, maintain.
	Fall 2009	The same test and benchmark was used.	Benchmark was met, maintain.
	Fall 2010	The same test and benchmark was used. 80% of the learners achieved 75%.	Faculty agreed to review of teaching/learning activities in courses with critical thinking outcomes.

Nursing faculty have the major responsibility for collecting, organizing, and reporting data. It must be done on a continuous basis. Setting up a process to record the information needed for systematic program evaluation is vital (Anema, Brown, & Stringfield, 2003). Table 17.3 provides examples.

APPROACHES TO REPORTING PROGRAM AND COURSE OUTCOMES

All systematic evaluation plans yield a great deal of information that is used in different ways. So, decisions must be made. Reports related to program and course outcomes are prepared with different levels of information and for diverse audiences. Reports, developed to present the program outcome information, include the following areas; what did you do, why did you do it, what did you find, and how will you use it? (Western Washington University, 2011). Consider the audience for a report and determine what they want to know. Audiences include accrediting bodies, state/federal agencies, external funding agencies, administrators, curriculum committees, alumni, and prospective students (Western Washington University, 2011).

By knowing the information above, it is possible to create appropriate reports. Informal reports may just highlight selected outcomes that are used for press releases and marketing bullet points. This is a positive way to share good news, both internally and externally. Formal reports are comprehensive and include details of each outcome, with appendices that provide supporting data in charts, tables, and examples from the primary data collected. Executive reports are short summaries of the information needed by the audience and are about one page long.

EXAMPLES OF DEVELOPMENT, MAINTENANCE, OR REVISION

- Additional program outcomes are developed to meet the **revised** accreditation standards that include global health content.
- A plan is **developed** to include the new requirement for a program exit standardized examination.
- The NCLEX-RN licensing examination pass rate is at 97%, which is 10% above the national average. That rate will be **maintained** for the program.
- The attrition rate for the program is less than the institution and national standards. That rate will be **maintained** for the program.
- The benchmark was to have 90% of the faculty hold doctoral degrees in the undergraduate program. The institutional and national requirements for similar programs with clinical components are 80%. The benchmark will be **revised** to 85%, which is above the standards.

- The number of credit hours allowed for undergraduate programs has been reduced from 130 hours to 120. **Revisions** will be made to the curriculum to meet that requirement.

EXAMPLES OF PROGRAM EVALUATION REPORTS

- Program faculty report describes current status of curriculum and how the outcome results support the need for improvement in certain areas.
- Admission marketing reports include student satisfaction highlights, how the mission to have excellent educational outcomes is achieved, retention rates, and faculty professional achievements in the different programs.
- A board of trustees report includes an executive summary of the program outcomes based on changes from the previous report.
- Outcomes that have not achieved identified goals can be used to gain additional resources (faculty, equipment, etc.) in the next budget cycle.
- Reports for external accrediting and regulatory agencies identify the specific information required and expect that the data are trended over time (attrition and graduation rates, pass rates on licensing and certification examinations, student demographics, faculty degrees, financial condition of an institution, comparison of resource allocations between programs, library holdings, etc.) (Western Washington University, 2011).

References

American Association of Colleges of Nursing. (2008). *Essentials series*. Retrieved November 1, 2011, from http://www.aacn.nche.edu/education-resources/essential-series

Anema, M. G., Brown, B. E., & Stringfield, Y. N. (2003). Organizing and presenting program outcome data. *Nursing Education Perspectives, 24*(6), 306–310.

Anema, M. G., & McCoy, J. (2010). *Competency-based nursing education: Guide to achieving outstanding learner outcomes*. New York, NY: Springer Publishing Company.

Billings, D. M., & Halstead, J. A. (2008). *Teaching in nursing: A guide for faculty*. St. Louis, MO: Elsevier-Saunders.

Bloom, B. S. (1956). *Handbook I: Taxonomy of educational objectives, the cognitive domain*. New York, NY: David McKay.

Commission on Collegiate Nursing Education. (2009). *Standards, procedures, and resources*. Retrieved November 1, 2011, from http://www.aacn.nche.edu/ccne-accreditation/standards-procedures-resources/overview

Cuevas, U. M., Matveev, A. G., & Miller, K. O. (2010). Mapping general education outcomes in the major: Intentionality and transparency. *Peer Review, 12*(1), 10–15.

Duignan, P. (2009). *What are outcomes systems?* Retrieved December 1, 2011, from http://knol.google.com/k/what-are-outcomes-systems#

Harden, R. M. (2001). AMEE Guide No. 21: Curriculum mapping: A tool for transparent and authentic teaching and learning. *Medical Teacher, 23*(2), 123–137.

Iwasiw, C., Goldenberg, D., & Andrusyszyn, M. (2009). *Curriculum development in nursing education.* Sudbury, MA: Jones and Bartlett.

Jabareen, Y. (2009). Building a conceptual framework: Philosophy, definitions, and procedure. *International Journal of Qualitative Methods, 8*(4), 49–62.

Keating, S. B. (2006). *Curriculum development and evaluation in nursing.* Philadelphia, PA: Lippincott Williams & Wilkins.

Keating, S. B. (2010). *Curriculum development and evaluation in nursing.* Philadelphia, PA: Lippincott Williams & Wilkins.

Leischow, S. J., & Milstein, B. (2006). Systems thinking and modeling for public health practice. *American Journal of Public Health, 96*(3), 403–405.

Lowenstein, A. J., & Bradshaw, M. J. (2007). *Fuszard's innovative teaching strategies in nursing and related health professions.* Sudbury, MA: Jones & Bartlett.

Meacham, J. (2008). What's the use of a mission statement? *Academe, 94*(1), 21–24.

National Association for Practical Nurse Education and Service, Inc. (2007). *Standards of practice and educational competencies of graduates of practical/vocational nursing programs.* Retrieved November 1, 2011, from http://www.napnes.org/about/standards/standards_read_only.pdf

National Council of State Boards of Nursing. (2011). *Find your state board of nursing.* Retrieved November 1, 2011, from https://www.ncsbn.org/2715.htm

National League for Nursing Accrediting Commission, Inc. (2008). *NLNAC accreditation manual.* Retrieved November 1, 2011, from http://nlnac.org/manuals/Manual2008.htm

National League for Nursing Accrediting Commission, Inc. (2011). *Guidelines for the preparation of the self-study report.* Retrieved November 1, 2011, from http://www.nlnac.org/resources/GuidelinesSSR.htm

National Organization for Associate Degree Nursing. (2006). *Position statement.* Retrieved November 1, 2011, from https://www.noadn.org/component/option,com_docman/Itemid,250/task,doc_view/gid,16

Nursing Management. (2010). *Mission, vision, values, objectives and philosophy of an organization.* Retrieved November 9, 2011, from http://currentnursing.com/nursing_management/mission_vision_values_of_organizations.html

Rogers, E. (1983). *Diffusion of innovations.* New York, NY: Free Press.

Trochim, W. M., Cabrera, D. A., Milstein, B., Gallagher, R. S., & Leischow, S. J. (2006). Practical challenges of systems thinking and modeling in public health. *American Journal of Public Health, 96*(3), 538–546.

Western Washington University, Center for Instructional Innovation and Assessment. (2011). *Comprehensive plans and information.* Retrieved October 30, 2011, from http://pandora.cii.wwu.edu/cii/resources/outcomes/program_assessment.asp

Wittmann-Price, R. A., & Fasolka, B. J. (2010). Objectives and outcomes: The fundamental difference. *Nursing Education Perspectives, 31*(4), 233–236.

Index